RUTH FIELD

is no professional fitness guru. She is, however, a devoted runner who, while pregnant with twins and under doctor's orders not to run, decided to write this book as an outlet for her frustration. She never dreamed anyone would actually read it. Let alone buy it.

THE GRIT DOCTOR

is not a fitness expert, nor is she a real doctor. Her profession is simply *grit,* but in this area she is, without question, the world's leading authority. The exercise routines in this book are intended for those in reasonable physical and mental health. If you have a genuine medical condition or underlying injury, are pregnant, or have any other health concerns (including past or current experience with an eating disorder), please consult your doctor before starting out. However, under no circumstances invent health concerns or problems and use them as an excuse to avoid running sessions.

THE EXPERIMENT

BECAUSE EVERY BOOK IS A TEST OF NEW IDEAS

RUTH FIELD AKA THE GRIT DOCTOR

GET OFF YOUR ASS AND RUN!

A TOUGH-LOVE RUNNING PROGRAM FOR LOSING THE EXCUSES *AND* THE WEIGHT

THE EXPERIMENT
NEW YORK

The Experiment, LLC
260 Fifth Avenue
New York, NY 10001-6408
theexperimentpublishing.com

This book contains the opinions and ideas of its author. It is intended to provide helpful and informative material on the subjects addressed in the book. It is sold with the understanding that the author and publisher are not engaged in rendering medical, health, or any other kind of personal professional services in the book. Please consult with your physician or other health care professional before beginning any diet or health program. The author and publisher specifically disclaim all responsibility for any liability, loss, or risk—personal or otherwise—that is incurred as a consequence, directly or indirectly, of the use and application of any of the contents of this book.

The Experiment's books are available at special discounts when purchased in bulk for premiums and sales promotions as well as for fundraising or educational use. For details, contact us at info@theexperimentpublishing.com.

Library of Congress Cataloging-in-Publication Data

Field, Ruth.
Get off your ass and run! : a tough-love running program for losing the excuses and the weight / by Ruth Field.
    p. cm.
    "First published in the United Kingdom in 2012 as Run Fat Bitch Run by Sphere, an imprint of Little, Brown Book Group."
    ISBN 978-1-61519-077-5 (pbk.)--ISBN 978-1-61519-170-3 (ebook) 1. Exercise for women. 2. Reducing exercises. I. Title.
    GV482.F5 2012
    613.7'12--dc23
                        2012036622

ISBN 978-1-61519-077-5
Ebook ISBN 978-1-61519-170-3

Cover design by Lindsey Andrews
Cover image of lying-down silhouette © iStockphoto | 4x6
Cover image of sitting silhouette © iStockphoto | 4x6
Cover image of running silhouette © iStockphoto | AF-studio
Text design by Pauline Neuwirth, Neuwirth & Associates, Inc.

Manufactured in the United States of America
Distributed by Workman Publishing Company, Inc.
Distributed simultaneously in Canada by Thomas Allen and Son Ltd.

First published April 2013
10 9 8 7 6 5 4 3 2 1

for Olly

Contents

PART 3 NOW WHAT?

GET OFF YOUR ASS AND *RUN!*

Who Is the Grit Doctor?

I am the Grit Doctor. I am a ruthless, no-nonsense motivator who will force you to do the things you don't want to do—in this case, run. I will bully you into submission and then inspire you to heights greater than you thought possible. I am the voice you will tune in to when you are feeling at your most lazy and inefficient and the one who will help you ignore the deafening call of the sofa. I will whisper in your ear, "Do you *really* need that?" when you are contemplating one more potato chip. I am the voice you need to listen to and obey.

Once you learn to understand and enjoy the voice of the Grit Doctor, it won't be long before you can tune in to it whenever you choose. The Grit Doctor will push you forward when you might otherwise give up. The voice of the Grit Doctor is what you've been missing in your life. You just didn't know it until now.

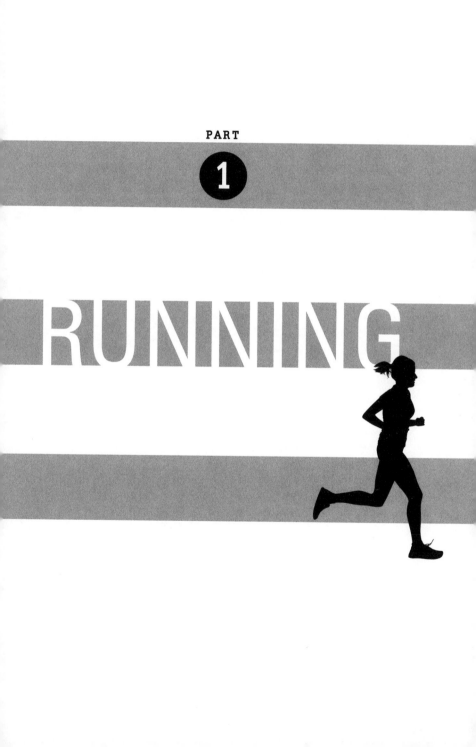

PART

1

RUNNING

Introduction

This book is not for the committed fitness freak. Nor is it meant for the super-motivated. I am not here to help you to run a marathon or sculpt your deltoids. If you already have the body you want—and that includes those of you who are fat and blissfully happy just as much as the super-slim and toned among you—congratulations. You don't need to read any further.

This book is specifically designed for those of you who are *unhappy with your body*. Those of you who feel stuck and unable to commit to any kind of exercise or diet for long enough to see any results. It is designed to shake you out of your complacence, get you up off the sofa, and make you embrace a new way of being.

The good news is that nothing in this book is rocket science. In fact, a great deal of it is common sense. *So why do I need to read it, then?* I hear you ask. Well, knowing something is common sense is all well and good, but when it is buried under layers of self-delusion, it's not always that easy to act on. You know that eating healthily is common sense, too, don't you? And yet that cake makes you drool with desire and you happily bypass the fruit bowl to get at it. So don't be fooled into thinking you know it all already. You don't.

When I say it's not rocket science, what I really mean is that if you're looking for the latest high-tech, Gwyneth Paltrow–approved weight-loss program, you've come to the wrong place. This book follows a basic formula: run, eat less junk, lose weight. Simple. But don't confuse simple with easy. Straightforward, yes. Easy, no.

Running is simple in the sense that it is entirely natural and instinctive. All able-bodied people were born to run. Just watch the way that any child, freed from the protective grasp of a parent's hand, joyfully runs about with complete and utter abandon. Nothing could be more natural. But while it is a simple activity, *easy* it isn't. Certainly not when you're doing it as a self-conscious adult as opposed to during a game of tag on the school playground. So in order to rediscover this natural gift that you were born with, you will need education, discipline, and commitment. But don't panic, the Grit Doctor will be with you all the way and will help you dig deep and find all three.

Before we get under way, there are three concepts you must take on board. Immediately.

1. **You need to be taught how to run.** It is not quite as simple as merely going outside and giving it a whirl.
2. When it comes to food and weight loss, the bottom line is this: **Your run will be your diet.** Quite literally.

And most important,

3. In order to hear my message clearly, and appreciate its value, **you will need to make friends with your inner bitch.** My own inner bitch is the Grit Doctor, and I'm lending her to you for the duration of this book. I hope you will come to know and love her and, ultimately, adopt her, adapt her, and make her your own.

Now I know that this whole Grit Doctor thing is in danger of making me sound like some kind of nut, but really I am just naming that voice we all have inside our heads. Yours may be lying dormant or suffocating under your excess weight, but *it is there.* That nagging little voice that makes you feel just a tad uncomfortable about helping yourself to another cookie or ignoring the wet laundry in order to watch one more episode of *Glee.* You know, the one you usually ignore. Well, not anymore. One of the things I am going to try to help you do is to listen much more carefully to that voice—amplify it, actually—until it really gets in your face.

The Grit Doctor will be with you throughout this book. She'll be there, holding up a mirror when you slump back onto the sofa, sighing that this all sounds too much like hard work and reaching for the chocolate. She will motivate, inspire, and, yes, even bully you into making the necessary changes in your life. Sometimes you will hate her. In fact, you may always hate her, but one day you'll want to shout back and show her who's boss. And when that happens, you'll know you've turned a corner. You've found your own inner bitch.

If tapping into this pool of negativity seems odd, or even unhealthy, let me say this by way of reassurance. The Grit Doctor is a *device* I have harnessed to help motivate myself to do the things I'd often really rather not. She is there only when I need her. I can say with absolute certainty that if I employed Grit Doctor tactics in all areas of my life *all of the time*, I would be extremely unpopular and probably divorced. But here's the thing: I know that with the Grit Doctor's help I can power through the boring bits of life with relative ease.

So I'm sure you've figured out by now that the Grit Doctor is not going to dress this up as "fun" and make you feel good about yourself if there's plainly nothing to feel good about. I don't want to waste my energy or yours filling your head with nonsense about how much fun running is and how great you look. The former is a lie, and the fact that you are reading this book ought to give you a clue about the latter. I want you to be honest with yourself, even hard on yourself, because there is no magic pill and none of it is easy. *Stop wanting things to be easy.* Once you accept—and I mean *really* accept—that life is not easy, it actually becomes a lot more manageable because you stop resisting the hard work and find the determination and grit that is required in order to achieve anything worthwhile. This is going to be hard. *But*—and this is the crucial BUT—**you are going to start *enjoying* hard. Embracing hard. Hard is going to be the new black.**

Once you have "got it" and achieved your desired weight, you will only need to find three 45-minute free periods each week in order to look great and eat well *for the rest of your life*. And you will have it forever and *wherever* you find yourself: on vacation, in the countryside, in the city, at your mom's, or on your way back from work, because it only involves putting on your shoes and stepping outside for 45 minutes. No fancy equipment, no having to get yourself somewhere else first, negotiating your way through rush-hour traffic or public transportation. You are *always* only two minutes away from getting the job done—two minutes spent putting on your sneakers and getting out of the front door, which is 90 percent of the battle WON.

THE *Grit Doctor* SAYS

OK, BITCHES. Let's get moving.

FAST TRACK OR SLOW COACH?

Some of you will find this easier than others. Perhaps the seed of motivation to get fit or lose weight has already been sown and is just waiting for a big bang to bring it to life. So if you're already feeling inspired and want to take the **Fast Track**, just jump ahead to page 47, where you'll find a simple step-by-step guide to getting started—far be it from me to hold you back if you're already raring to go. And you can always come back and read the other bits later.

But for those of you who quite literally need dragging out from under the blanket, the **Slow Coach** approach is tailor-made for you. Don't be embarrassed—the fact that you've bought this book is a step in the right direction, and you'll be up and running in no time at all. You'll probably need to read everything straight through, including the more detailed beginners' program designed specifically for chronic couch potatoes. The Grit Doctor is not shy of hand-holding and will walk you through all the necessary steps. You may start off as a Slow Coach and discover midway through that you want to Fast Track or vice versa. This is also fine.

#gritdoctor

GET OFF YOUR ASS AND RUN!

Ruth . . .

I STARTED RUNNING when I was twenty-four. I'd given up all exercise sometime during college, having previously been really into sports, and I knew that something was missing from my life. I was also single again after a long relationship, so maybe that had something to do with it, too.

I had begun my apprenticeship as an attorney, and my adviser insisted on eating a proper lunch on a daily basis, by which I mean some Chinese or something equally naughty and spectacularly calorific. Bless him, it was the only meal of the day that he "took," as he would say. Unfortunately, my eating habits soon spiraled out of control as I continued to eat a huge evening meal and a hearty breakfast without doing any exercise at all except running to and from court. I immediately started to pile on the pounds. (Someone recently pointed out to me that I have never been fat, and I think it is only fair to own up to this. I have never been overweight in the strictest sense of the word. But, like most women, there have been times in my life when I have definitely needed to lose a few pounds, and this was one of them. I was fifteen pounds over my usual weight, my clothes were getting really tight, and when I looked in the mirror I saw the makings of a very fat bitch indeed.)

It was around this time that a great friend of mine, Jane—who was not known for her athletic prowess—announced in the pub that she was going to run the London Marathon. I was stunned, as were all our friends. Jane was comfortably the least likely of all of us to do something like this, which of course made her announcement all the more impressive. I was beside myself with envy and immediately said I would run with her (mainly to impress everyone else), having no idea how to run or what a marathon was all about.

I had six months to figure it out. What kept me going in those early days was the knowledge that I couldn't back out after making such a public proclamation. I was fully committed to running the marathon, and quitting was *not an option*. And I knew I didn't have a hope in hell if I didn't start training.

I can honestly say I hated every single one of those early runs. I was shocked at how hard it was and ashamed at how unfit I had become as I struggled to run for even five minutes without feeling like I was on the verge of a heart attack. It was incredibly difficult and not helped by the dreadful route I chose—laps of Clapham Common, a flat and featureless landscape that left me feeling totally uninspired. It didn't occur to me to get a book on running or to ask for help. I just kept at it, with the Grit Doctor always breathing down my neck, telling me that if I didn't get it together I'd be a total loser and that Jane would beat me. Which she did, by the way. (Ten years later and it still pains me to acknowledge that!)

So that's how it started. I had needed to do something to burn off those lunches and then, by pure coincidence one day, my competitive spirit was reawakened. I had no idea at the time what a great, lifelong gift Jane and my adviser had indirectly given me. I had no intention of becoming a runner; I just wanted to lose some weight, run this race, and then get back to my normal life. What I didn't know then was how running would ultimately transform so many other areas of my life. No longer would I need to complain about the cost of a gym membership or find time to join a class—and actually attend. I would have something to do all by myself for the rest of my life. Something that would satisfy me completely.

There was never one moment for me when it all "clicked." There was just before and after I ran. I only truly became a runner *after* that first marathon, because beforehand I really hated it: the training, the stress, the knowledge that I wasn't nearly fit enough, and the constant nagging feeling that I might not do myself justice. I certainly wasn't planning on running *ever again* after the marathon. And I didn't run for a couple of weeks once it was over. I couldn't anyway—my toes were covered in blisters. But to my surprise, I found myself really missing how running had made me feel. I suddenly felt the urge to go out for a run. I dug out my sneakers and hit the park, and that was the moment that really marked the beginning of my life as a runner—it felt like I was choosing to get out there in a way I hadn't before. So having thought I wouldn't ever want to run again, I soon found I couldn't live without it.

THE *grit doctor* SAYS

YOU MAY NEVER actually enjoy running. If you are one of the lucky ones, you will reach a stage during some runs when everything feels so right that you almost forget you are running. You are running "in the zone," and that is a real pleasure. But it doesn't always happen, and it doesn't always last. You will hate some runs from start to finish. What you *enjoy* is less the run itself and more what the practice of running is enabling you to do in the rest of your life. The pleasure you really get from running is *from the fact that you have run*—that you put your sneakers on, braved the great outdoors, and actually did it, in spite of all the excuses you could think of not to.

Running requires effort every time. It is very important to understand and accept this at the start to avoid unnecessary disappointment and motivation meltdown.

THE OFFICIAL PRE-RUNNING FAT ASS PLEDGE

I, _____, do solemnly declare and accept that I am a FAT ASS and I want to do something about it. I promise not to waste any more valuable fat-busting time buying fancy equipment, joining expensive gyms and exercise classes, or filling in charts with weights and measurements. I will no longer be seduced by fad diets. I will stop making excuses for myself and, holding hands with my inner bitch, I will haul my fat ass off the sofa and get out of the front door.

I swear on my mother's life to do as the Grit Doctor tells me and at all times to retain my sense of humor.

Signed: _____

Dated: _____

Getting Shit Done

Running makes you rich. . . .

Well, not exactly. What I mean is that it is a very cheap hobby. In fact, it is essentially totally free, requiring no financial investment on your part. Other than the cost of the occasional new pair of sneakers, it does not involve spending money on fancy new clothes, equipment, or expensive membership fees. You can even run without shoes if you have to; indeed, running barefoot on a beautiful beach at sunrise is to be recommended at least once in your life. Plus, running is a natural performance enhancer. Your time spent running can be used for quiet meditation or for your most powerful and creative thinking, making you an all-around more efficient operator, which will lead to you being more effective at work. And being more effective will probably lead to making more money—in the long run (pun intended).

MAKE A LIST of all the things you have promised to do when you are thin.

For example:

When I am thin, I will . . .

☐ Have more sex

☐ Apply for my dream job

☐ Sign up for a charity 5K and actually *run* it

☐ Ask out the hot barista in Starbucks

☐ Go on a beach vacation without having to cover up

☐ Marry Ryan Gosling/Jessica Alba

The Grit Doctor is not a fan of lists—they are, quite frankly, a waste of time that would be better spent actually *doing* the stuff on the list. (No, you don't need to write something down in order to know that you need to do it. Put down your pen. Now.) The point of this exercise is extremely important. NOW THAT YOU HAVE WRITTEN YOUR "WHEN I AM THIN" LIST, RIP IT UP AND THROW IT AWAY. GIVE UP TO-DO LISTS. TAKE UP *GETTING SHIT DONE*.

"When I am thin, I will . . ." is one of the biggest and most dangerous delusions out there. It is, in fact, keeping you fat. Thin doesn't just happen, and it certainly doesn't just happen if you have been overweight for a long time. It is extremely difficult, not to mention monstrously dull, committing to diet after diet in an attempt to lose weight.

How many times have you started a diet before? Be honest.

How many Mondays started out with the best of intentions? Drinking gallons of water, eating rice cakes and apples, feeling vaguely faint by going-home time, getting to about Wednesday and then caving in and eating a slice of cake? OK, maybe you managed a few weeks before the cake eating began, but eventually those weeks of good behavior were completely wasted. Or maybe you lost twenty pounds on a great diet, but over the rest of the year it crept back on, and when you weighed yourself after the holidays, what do you know? Back to square one. *I know it is hard.* Losing weight is really, really hard, especially if you are going about it in the "dieting" way.

The thing is, you have almost certainly set yourself impossibly high standards when it comes to the size and weight you need to be before you can do and have all the things on your "when I am thin" list. The idea that when you are thin you will be able to do *x*, *y*, and *z*—including exercising—is actually a major factor in keeping the weight on. The fear that you *can't* do something because you are overweight is paralyzing.

The only way to lose weight effectively and forever is through a committed exercise routine and, through that, *changing your attitude toward food*. **Exercise is the real key to weight loss, not food.** The whole concept of a diet is that it has an end point: "Lose X pounds in X number of weeks!" It is all a complete lie. It is almost impossible to lose weight permanently through dieting, because when the diet ends you go back to what you ate before and the weight creeps back on. Crash diets are even worse. Losing an enormous amount of weight in a short space of time for a special occasion puts your body and mind under great strain, and you'll revert back to your old ways as soon as the wedding/vacation/high school reunion outfit comes off.

Starting a diet—even a good one—is a very difficult way to solve any weight issue because it addresses only one factor inside an enormously intricate problem. Don't get me wrong, what you are eating is undoubtedly part of the issue, but it is *only part of it*. I'm no psychologist, but it's well known that eating is a very emotional thing. Your reasons for eating, your state of mind, your happiness levels, your body's learned expectation of what you are going to put into it, your ideas about what it means to be hungry or thirsty, when and how you feel satisfied, and your bad habits all contribute to what you put in your mouth. Trying to turn yourself into a rice-cake-munching waif on a Monday morning when up until Sunday night you have been used to pizza and Sour Patch Kids is going to be impossible for your confused body. You will feel faint and weird and just plain starving hungry, and will inevitably fall off the wagon.

THE grit Doctor SAYS

STOP FEELING DEPRESSED about being fat and start doing something about it. Go outside and start walking.

Throw away the diet books. For the moment, you can keep the contents of your fridge and cupboards and continue to eat in exactly the same way as you always have. Your current eating habits are not important—they are entirely secondary and **much less** **critical** than getting you outside and running. It is vital to your success not to do too many things at once. So your priority right now, your **only** priority, is running. Focus all your energy on this one thing—not new clothes, new sneakers, new body, new you, new anything. Forget buying anything new, and just use what you have for the moment. Get yourself outdoors and start moving. That is all you need to do to start losing weight. Keep the rest of your life the same for now and simply concentrate on getting the hang of the basics of running. I know this is hard, but it is not as hard as buying, preparing, cooking, and eating three restricted diet meals a day and spending at least 50 percent of the rest of the day fantasizing about what you would rather be eating. I reckon that must take up a good few hours of your day at least. And it is all time wasted.

Learning to run, on the other hand, is an hour and a half a day, tops. I know that sounds like a lot, but it's an investment and I promise that you won't regret it. Plus, it acts as fitness time but also diet time, and there are a million tangential benefits that will come from the latter. For you Slow Coaches, that means you get a whole lot more bang for your buck.

THE *grit doctor* SAYS

YOU MAY BE feeling an urge to get started. If so, you must capitalize on this immediately and skip to the Six-Step Program in Chapter 3 (page 47) and begin Step 1 without further ado. YOU DO NOT NEED TO DO ANYTHING ELSE FIRST. You can always read the preceding chapters on the toilet or in the bath after you've completed Step 1. The Grit Doctor is eager for you to take advantage of any motivation you have as it arises. Go on then, get cracking.

For the rest of you, read on.

RUNNING IS THE ANSWER

Forget all that Pilates, yoga, Zumba, even gym sessions. Forget all of it. You will never have the body you want, nor the mental strength and stamina required to maintain it, until you understand and practice that **running is the answer**. It is the only answer. No exceptions. Ah, I hear you object, what about so-and-so and so-and-so who have perfect physiques and are not runners? Well, I'm not talking to a professional gymnast or ballet dancer, am I? And trust me, they all know the value of what I am telling you. All other exercise, at the level at which you are doing it, is invariably *less* than running. By which I mean it is not enough. Not enough to change you and your body in the sort of permanent way I have in mind. And so for the purposes of this book, ladies and gentlemen, lolling around on a Pilates ball or flexing your nonexistent biceps in the mirror doesn't count. Give it all up and devote yourself entirely to the practice of running for now.

Once you have mastered the art of running, you can add in a spot of yoga or indeed any sport to your fitness regimen, although I recommend that you make it *as well as* rather than *instead of* running. But give it all up for now until you have "got" running and are fully committed to its practice. Of course, if you work out religiously at the gym five times a week every week (and spend that time actually exercising and not fumbling around with equipment and ogling other people's bodies), you will get fit. But I am addressing those of you who remain overweight and can't understand why when you are attending an aerobics class twice a week or playing flag football on the weekend. You are simply not doing anywhere near enough fat-busting, cardiovascular exercise to change anything about your body and your weight. Forget about classes and designer sports gear and all the time-wasting that surrounds them. Do something more effective, something more strenuous, something that will really, *really* burn away the excess flab—in a way and at a rate that nothing you have tried thus far has been able to.

WHY RUN?

Now, why is it that running is the answer? Well, it is different from all other forms of exercise, at the level at which you are doing them, because *it is much harder*—not harder as in more complicated but harder as in more physically strenuous. And because it is that much harder, ultimately it is that much more rewarding, both in terms of the dramatic physical changes to your body and indeed to your life in general. You only have to ask any of your friends who run regularly or look at the lean, mean body of any long-distance runner to see why. Running requires discipline and commitment above and beyond other forms of exercise. It all has to come from you. There is no help or encouragement to be gleaned from an instructor or classmate, no underfloor heating or delicate scent of incense, and no one but yourself to get you motivated or to blame if you fail. The first 10 minutes or so of each run are hellish *every* time. You are entirely at the mercy of the elements; there are no breaks midway through, no variation in the movement, no halftime snacks, and no team banter. Running is the ultimate physical challenge because, at first glance, it looks boring, repetitive, difficult, relentless, punishing, and joyless. **Sounds fun? Ha. I told you it was hard, but remember, hard is going to be the *new black*.**

But surely there's an easier way?

THE *Grit Doctor* SAYS

THERE ISN'T. The Grit Doctor would like to remind you—*again*—that embracing the fact that this is going to be hard is the only cure for the terminally unmotivated. The Grit Doctor suspects that you have become an expert at avoiding the hard things in life. You find yourself stuck in an exercise/weight rut from which you seem unable to escape and cannot understand why your lame efforts fail to yield spectacular results. You have come to expect that somehow you will get thin or fit "the easy way" and keep starting a Pilates class or making it to the swimming pool once a month. You think that this is sufficient effort on your part. It isn't.

Look on the bright side, once you choose to follow the Grit Doctor and surrender to the idea that it will be hard, the world becomes your oyster. Hard is no longer something that you studiously avoid but instead something that you know is necessary to get the results you so desperately want. All the clichés back me up:

> The *harder* the challenge, the sweeter the victory.
> The *harder* the conflict, the more glorious the triumph.

The good news is that once you have become a runner (and that does not mean once you have been on your first run—you *become a runner* when you have been at it for some time, when you are several months into running regularly), it's only a matter of time before you no longer find it hard. Ultimately, you will need to create new levels of hard in order to challenge and stretch yourself further, and you will come to enjoy this process. For now, just accept that running is hard and you are probably not going to enjoy it. But believe that there must be something in it—something pretty special. Otherwise why are the parks and streets filled with runners at all times of the day and night as they keep coming back for more?

THE *Grit Doctor* SAYS

SPECTACULAR RESULTS ARE only achieved through spectacular effort. No exceptions.

Perhaps a few of you have been totally put off by some of the points raised above. And maybe you have been running a couple of times in the past and decided it is actually unbelievably boring, you got nothing out of it, and you vowed never to do it again. Be honest, though: Have you dismissed other forms of exercise after trying them just once or twice? Have you *ever* been the weight you want to be? No, that doesn't include when you were a toddler or, in fact, any prepuberty age.

THE grit doctor SAYS

THERE ARE NO shortcuts, and by perpetually looking for them you are wasting valuable time.

This is, in many ways, about changing your mind-set. Your success—particularly in these areas you have been struggling with—depends on it. Assume it is going to be hard, a bit mentally and physically painful, challenging on all sorts of levels, and involving some sacrifices, albeit only of the "giving up the TV and sofa for an hour" variety. I'm afraid that in order to even begin to enjoy running and its numerous benefits, you have to commit to practicing it regularly over a long period of time. It doesn't work any other way.

You must have some friends or work colleagues who run or, at the very least, be acquainted with at least a few running nuts. Think about them for a few minutes. Think of their physique and eating habits. Are those runners total losers? Fat, lazy, and woefully ineffective at work? I didn't think so. Now ask yourself, are they fitter, more toned, and healthier than you? Are they generally more positive, more proactive, more efficient operators? Do the runners tend to get things done, do what they say they are going to do, and exercise a certain discipline in other areas of their life? Do they seem to be able to get more done with less fuss? If, as I suspect, the answer to at least some of these questions is yes, running is the reason why.

Every day was a different run. But the one constant through it all was that for the first twelve minutes of every run I just wanted to stop. I would rather be doing anything else. As I pulled on my socks at 6 a.m. in the dark or during the first few yards on the pavement or when my lungs filled with cold air and said, "Oh no, not this again," I would be wishing I was back in bed, at work, on the beach, out with friends, reading a book, watching TV—anything but this. My knees were saying, "Really?," my hamstrings were tightening, my mind was telling me to walk, and I had an overall sensation that everything was about to break with a massive ping.

And then, as if out of nowhere, I would introduce myself to myself. My breathing would regulate, my muscles would soften and warm, my heart would beat and chime "good morning," my feet would find a rhythm, and I would feel, see, hear, and BE my body. And this happened every day I ran. Every day I would overcome the obstacle of myself—my motivation, my physical ailments—and win. Every day I ran I would win. Even if it was a bad run, it was a bad run out of the way—which was a win.

After a while this gives you such confidence—a new and positive outlook. You teach yourself that you will overcome any obstacle if you put the effort in. Small win after small win, day after day. If you put the effort in you win. No matter what happens during the day or what you have to face—if you run you win. I started taking that into other areas of my life. Things got done in areas where they hadn't before. More

#gritdoctor GET OFF YOUR ASS AND RUN!

time was given to quality work, daunting tasks didn't seem so daunting, and I was able to prioritize very effectively.

So my body became my body; the more I ran the more it became mine. It slimmed down, it strengthened, it shed excess, it felt good, and it craved good things. I ate differently as my body demanded it—a diet I had never eaten before, a healthy diet, and I kept hydrated. My skin changed—softer, clearer. But the food was the major transformation. Good fuel food 80 percent of the time and then 20 percent of the time I ate and enjoyed whatever I wanted and it didn't matter.

Mentally I was clearer. I would leave the office with a jumble of thoughts from the day and over the period of my run home the irrelevant ones were stripped away and I was left with the important things to focus on. Problems would get solved so the stress would disappear and I would be left with what was important—invariably my husband and children. ■

MAKE RUNNING YOUR RELIGION

There is an obvious connection between lack of motivation to exercise and general disarray in other areas of your life. This is every runner's secret: Running is the key to successful living. By *successful* I simply mean living your life the way you choose to and being able to enjoy it fully.

It is the practice of running that enables the rest of the runner's life to progress that much more effectively. Just speak to your runner friends and listen to them go on about how their lives have changed since they took up running. Anyone who has run a marathon will tell you that it really does take you to a whole new level of being and operational efficiency. In order to have the body you want, you need to make running your religion. It is, in fact, much

GETTING SHIT DONE

like the practice of religion in that it is *only* in the practicing of it that you receive its benefits. Knowing about it and trying it once or twice will reveal nothing to you. It is only through a committed routine over several weeks and months that the benefits become evident—slowly and surely. You will see improvements not just physically but in every area of your life, as well. And that lasts forever, or for as long as you choose to continue to practice.

Ruth . . .

MY HUSBAND, OLLY, and I were lucky enough to take a three-month honeymoon—the final stop of which was Perth, Australia, so I could meet Olly's totally gorgeous grandmother, then age ninety-three. Olly adored his grandmother, and it was very easy to see why when I met her for the first time. She clasped my face in her hands and said, "Well, hello, dear, I've been dying to meet you," and sat me down for a nice cup of tea—the first of many.

It was Christmas and we were coming to the end of our trip, but we had spent only a fraction of the money we had saved, such was the generosity and hospitality of Olly's family and friends in Australia. Throughout our trip Olly had been talking about this novel that he'd had in his head for the past decade. He had practically written it the way he spoke about it—he had all the characters' names and the locations for the story, the entire plot, and even the title. He seemed so keen to at least try to get this book onto the page. And so, in a moment of madness on New Year's Eve, we decided to resign from our jobs and take a further six months off to enable Olly to have a crack at writing. We posted our resignation letters on New Year's Day and then phoned our parents. Needless to say our "plan" went down like some-

GET OFF YOUR ASS AND RUN!

thing resembling a shit sandwich to everyone concerned, especially when it was followed, a few weeks later, with the news that we were expecting twins.

We suddenly had this huge stretch of time in front of us and felt incredibly overwhelmed and excited at the prospect of all the traveling we had left to do before the babies came. The book would get written while we moved from place to place in Southeast Asia, the idea being that that would be the best place to travel on what was now a very tight budget. But it turned out to be very difficult to write when we were moving around from country to country and hostel to hostel. Olly became adamant that he needed to be settled in one place for his creative juices to flow. Fair enough, I thought. Plus, I was desperate by now for some sort of settled routine and was dying to eat some of my own cooked food. It was with all this in mind that at an Internet café in Laos we decided upon France (the food was the deciding factor) and sent numerous e-mails to owners of vacation rentals. One was beyond our 600-euro-a-month maximum budget but looked so gorgeous—a bastide village house—that on a whim I e-mailed the owners. I told them we couldn't afford the advertised rent but that we could commit to four months and that my husband was writing a novel. The wonderful couple took pity on us and wrote back saying we could have it for 600 euro and that there was a lovely peaceful terrace and not one but two desks for Olly to write. The airport was close enough for me to get back to the UK with cheap flights if and when necessary. Clearly this was meant to be. So off to France we went.

I was in heaven when we arrived and I saw our kitchen—a huge farmhouse-style affair complete with modern appliances. My pregnancy cravings soon turned to pastry and all things French. Olly had brought an old copy of *Larousse Gastronomique* with us in the hope I would become some sort of Michelin-starred chef. I did learn a few tricks as I plowed my way through it and have, I like to think,

GET OFF YOUR ASS AND RUN!   #gritdoctor

perfected the art of the tarte tatin and the soufflé. The idea was that I was going to paint and cook while Olly wrote. So far, so good. But it wasn't long before we started to struggle. I had done about one pathetic sketch since arrival, and asking Olly for his word count was like poking a bear with a stick. With each passing day, fewer and fewer words got written.

I got this idea into my head that if Olly would just *run* he would be able to write so much more easily. I remembered how it had been such an effective tool for me when I was working, particularly when I had a difficult piece of written work to get done. I would always go running first, to think about what I was going to write, to order my thoughts and then to organize them on the page upon my return. It was *always* easier to do after a run and, invariably, better quality, too. I was under doctor's orders not to run, but I felt sure that if I could, I would also find painting easier. But I couldn't, so I didn't (pathetic excuse, I know). And that is how this book was born. Olly finally did what I had been telling him to do ever since we met: put on his sneakers and went outside for a run.

I make it sound easy when it was anything but. Poor Olly was very unfit, and I knew he was going to hate the walking, get bored, run too quickly and get all out of breath, then moan about it when he got home and probably never go again. So I briefed him on how to approach it—slowly, slowly, slowly. He did, to a certain extent, follow my instructions, and at least he didn't overdo it so much that he injured himself or put himself off for life. Not during his first few forays outside, anyway.

Bear in mind this is a man who had never failed to use any opportunity to adamantly reject running ever since we'd met two years before: "It's so boring," "I've always hated it," "I don't know why you bother," "I can't think of anything I'd rather do less." I certainly had my work cut out for me to get him going and try to keep him motivated. I hasten to add that he did not do this for me or for the book. I swear, after two years of watching how I eat and keep fit and focused, and listening to me drone on about where he was going wrong, he just woke up one morning and announced he was going for a run. I nearly fell off my chair. He probably just went to get an hour's peace and quiet away from me, but hey, whatever gets you out of the front door. (He also told me to stop carrying on about how great it is and write it all down instead. So here I am.) It was nothing short of a miracle. I truly believe that if he can do it, anyone can. And if I can convert him, I can convert anybody. Including you.

To: The Grit Doctor
From: Olly
Re: My First Run

The first five minutes felt pretty good. It was nearly all down-hill, following the road out of our little village and down toward the valley floor. With the wind in my hair, my belly giving me some momentum, and my legs finally starting to loosen up, I was beginning to think this might not be as bad as I'd feared. Then I hit the flat. Suddenly it didn't feel quite so straightforward anymore.

After about five minutes of gentle jogging, I slowed, slowed some more, and then came to a halt. But Ruth's advice kept ringing in my ears so I forced myself to keep walking, even if it was with my hands on my head while sucking in air. I then walked for about the next fifteen to twenty minutes, until breaking into another gentle jog. It didn't last long, and I quickly reverted to walking again. I tried very hard to appreciate the winter landscape around me: the leafless trees, the mud-brown fields, the fact that I wasn't at work. At the end of the circuit was a long section uphill back into the walled, bastide town. I walked the whole way up (hoping Ruth wasn't spying on me from some unseen position) until I hit the village square and then ran from there back to our house. I beat my hands on the door, sweat dripping down my face, until Ruth opened up and I fell inside. I felt bloody terrible. All in all I'd run about half a mile, and all of that downhill. I checked my belly just to see if it had decreased in size. There was a long, long way to go. ▪

#gritdoctor GET OFF YOUR ASS AND RUN!

Delusions of *Thinneur*

Running improves your sex life. . . .

There is no doubt that running improves the blood flow to your vital organs, giving you more energy and enthusiasm, if you get my drift. And if you are not getting any, running is a fantastic sex substitute—not only does the glow make you look as though you are getting plenty of action, but your relaxed and calm demeanor also makes you seem more like someone who is getting some than the wound-up, tense types about whom people always say, "He/she needs to get laid." You know who you are.

REACQUAINTING YOURSELF WITH YOUR INNER BITCH

The majority of us delude ourselves that we look a bit better than we actually do. A bit thinner, a bit hotter. We suck our stomachs in while in front of the mirror, preening and posing in a way that shows us in our very best light. Minus the double chin. With cheekbones. Our "mirror pose" bears no resemblance to how we actually appear to other people. We never display ourselves like that when walking about, at work talking to colleagues, or flirting in a bar. Occasionally you might catch yourself unaware in a mirror or a store window and recoil in horror at the stooped, tired, cheekboneless blob staring back at you. But you glance away quickly and stop off at the store on the way home for a bottle of wine and a king-size Snickers. Sound familiar?

THE *Grit Doctor* SAYS

STOP TELLING YOURSELF that you look great. You are robbing yourself of vital fuel required to kick-start yourself into action.

Try letting it all hang out, double chin included. Scrutinize yourself naked, and in the quest for a better, leaner body, tell yourself the ugly truth. Otherwise, if you constantly tell yourself you are looking good, you are denying yourself the catalyst required to improve those pudgy thighs and thick waistline.

NEGATIVE AFFIRMATIONS

When my little sister Anna was trying to lose a few pounds for a party and came to me for advice, it was with a degree of trepidation that I revealed to her my deepest, darkest dieting secret. When I want to lose a few pounds urgently, I look in the mirror early in the morning—pre-shower, no makeup, and with my entire naked body in view—and I repeat to myself over and over again, "You fat bitch." I then glance immediately at Cameron Diaz or another equally buff celeb in a bikini (*People* magazine's illuminating "Amazing Bodies" specials are perfect for this part of the exercise), and the mantra begins to take on a life of its own. My sister laughed a little anxiously at this apparently demented pearl of sisterly wisdom. "Try it out," I said, "and I bet your diet and exercise plan will be easier to follow. When you are tempted by something naughty for lunch, recall the images to mind—you versus Diaz—and repeat the mantra over and over again. I guarantee you will change your mind and go for the healthy option, and less of it."

Feel free to invent your own mantra that kick-starts you into action: "MAN UP!" "MOVE, YOU LAZY PIG!" Or any number of less aggressive options—provided they motivate you to get going.

To: The Grit Doctor
From: Anna
Re: Are You Mad?

When my sister gave me this dark and twisted advice to help me lose a few pounds for a party, my initial reaction was absolute horror. First, wasn't Ruth supposed to say, without hesitation, that I didn't need to lose any weight whatsoever? Second, isn't this sort of thing "thinspiration" and very unhealthy? Third, rather than calling myself a fat bitch, wasn't I meant to love my body blah blah blah? Anyway, knowing that my older sister can be slightly unorthodox, but as ever trusting her judgment, I did as I was told. I found a picture of Cameron Diaz running along the beach in a stringy white bikini—athletic, lean, happy, and healthy—and I stuck it to my bathroom mirror. Every morning when I got out of the shower, I stood naked in front of the mirror, looked at my body, looked at Cameron's, looked back at mine, and said to myself (out loud to make it more forceful—again on Ruth's advice), "YOU FAT BITCH!"

I don't really know exactly what it achieved psychologically, but it certainly made forgoing a morning croissant a lot easier. Thinking to myself *YOU FAT BITCH* and then averting my eyes as I went past the bakery on my morning walk to the station had me giggling to myself. When I went out running I would think of Cameron bounding down the beach and the image would spur me on.

Sure enough, by the time the party came around I felt fabulous. Loads of people commented that I looked great, and I found myself giggling once more as it hit me: there I was at the party—lean, happy, and healthy and feeling on top of the world. ▪

As the Grit Doctor made clear from the outset, it's all about channeling your inner bitch. Don't have one? Yes, you do. It's simply hidden under layer upon layer of soft, self-delusional, positive crap, which, luckily, is very easy to peel away. The next section will tell you how.

HOW TO CHANNEL YOUR INNER BITCH

Believe me when I say that we all have an inner bitch. In fact, I'd go so far as to argue that it's one of the things that makes us human. I bet you find it easy enough to tap into your nasty side when it's directed against others, don't you? Well, I want you to turn that judgmental, sharp-tongued bitch on yourself.

Close your eyes and take a deep breath. Bring to mind a work colleague or family member who really gets on your nerves. Focus on the specific quality or action that most incenses you about that person. Pause and contemplate the words and phrases that are now springing to mind quite effortlessly. *Voilà!* This is your nasty side. Congratulations. Isn't it amazing how loudly and clearly you can hear that voice when it is directed at others? OK, good. The key is to now turn your inner bitch against yourself. Say all those horrible things that sprang to mind moments ago, but this time *to yourself, about yourself.* Yes, YOU.

Think about the part of your body that you dislike the most. Really dwell on it for a few moments. Then think of the celebrity who is lucky enough to be in possession of the perfect example of that very body part.* Imagine kidnapping the celebrity and stealing those thighs/abs/biceps for yourself. Thy inner bitch shall covet Kristen Bell's ass.

---

*And remember, only a tiny proportion of the picture-perfect Hollywood A-list are the kind of genetic freaks who are actually born with the perfect set of long legs or pert derriere. They pay their own Grit Doctor–esque trainers to work them into submission. And they don't eat. And don't get me started on what is done to your average celeb before you see her on the front of your favorite magazine: hours (possibly days) spent in hair and makeup before a photo shoot, only for the one shot plucked from the billion taken to get Photoshopped to within an inch of its life. However, hot celebrities still look pretty good in the flesh, and they don't have the mirror-pose problem, so don't let all this cheer you up too much.

KEEP YOUR SENSE of humor at all times. You're going to need it.

Next time you're sitting on the sofa, watching some banal reality television program that you promised yourself you *would not watch tonight* so you could begin a new book/call your parents/clean out your closet, just pause and listen carefully for a moment. Can you hear a nagging little voice, like a mosquito buzzing around in your head? *I knew you wouldn't do it. I knew you would give up, I knew you would fail. No one is going to believe a word you say if you can't even stick to a small promise like not watching this garbage.* BINGO. That is your inner bitch.

Now that you have located that voice, you need to start becoming closer friends with it. Simply listen to it more often and imagine what it would say in certain situations. Answering to your inner bitch is the best exercise for strengthening your relationship. You are identifying and cultivating your nasty side and directing it against yourself to help you achieve success. The idea is not that you berate yourself to the point where the only reasonable response is to say, "I'm so depressed I want to bury myself in a mountain of potato chips." It should be more, "I am disgusted by this, and I am going to do something about it right now!" There is a clear distinction between the two. Be bold and assertive in the language you use, not wimpy and victim-esque. Remember, the point is to get you motivated to run, not to binge-eat yourself to death.

If you are struggling to locate your inner bitch, try this visualization technique: Close your eyes and take a deep breath. Imagine a terrifying bitch you sort of admire in real life (your old sports teacher from school, perhaps) or a fantasy bitch (Meryl Streep from *The Devil Wears Prada* is a good one) and have a pretend conversation with her. What would *she* say if she walked into your living room now and saw you slumped on the sofa?

Ruth . . .

THE IDEA OF calling myself a fat bitch and advising others to do the same is simply a device that I have found to be hilariously motivating. It is never supposed to savage our self-esteem, nor is it to be taken seriously except in the context of getting us into our sneakers—ideally, laughing—and out of the front door. I honestly find negative affirmations much more effective than their saccharine counterparts when it comes to getting me going. I think it's mainly because they make me laugh, although having said that, I always found the idea of positive affirmations pretty amusing. Looking in the mirror and repeating "I am beautiful and clean and pure and I deserve to be loved" or some other such nonsense—I could never take myself seriously. In fact, is it ever possible to take yourself seriously when you're talking to your reflection in a mirror?

The whole thing is just so unnatural. So if I'm going to do it, I find that calling myself nasty names is far more motivating, *and* it has the added benefit of really making me laugh.

Humor is a great motivational tool. Taking yourself too seriously can be paralyzing, and I find there's a huge release when I'm able to laugh at myself. We all automatically feel psychologically lighter when we laugh, and that somehow makes it easier to do things. That is my experience, and I realize that perhaps it's not for everyone, but my sister and I have conversations along these lines all the time and never fail to cheer each other up. And I'm sure we're not the only sisters who are brutally honest with each other. If one of us is really down about something, be it weight gain or a sudden outbreak of acne, the other never takes a light approach. It's much more likely to be along the lines of "Yes, you are a fat bitch—sort it out!," which instantly makes the other laugh and start to feel better and, crucially, motivated. In facing your fears, sharing them, and having them confirmed rather than batted away by a well-meaning friend ("No, you're not *fat*! You're curvy!"), you are bravely facing up to the truth. This allows you to do something about whatever it is that's making you unhappy. The minute a friend tells you what they think you want to hear, you go straight back to the sofa and your *Mad Men* box set, happily devour a tub of Phish Food, and remain safe in the knowledge that you're not fat, you're basically Christina Hendricks's doppelgänger. (You're not. *She* is curvy. *You* are fat.) But if you take matters in hand and run an eight-miler on a Sunday morning, you can eat that ice cream without a trace of guilt and probably have Don Draper afterward. On the other hand, if you're one of those guys letting your friends fool you into thinking you look like Don in a suit, this goes for you, too. Bros don't let bros get fat.

SEVEN KILLER EXCUSES

1. I don't have the right build for running.

There is no such thing as the right build for running. Any build will do. This excuse hides an underlying fear of failure. Hefty men and large-breasted ladies, in particular, are fond of this excuse. Well, I ran a race with an EE-cup lady friend. She wore two sports bras and had less nipple-chafing than I (a B-cup on a good day), *and* she beat me, so there!

To: The Grit Doctor
From: Alice
Re: Being Supportive

I didn't think I had the right frame for running. I had what is referred to as a "heavy frame" supporting an overly large chest that had been known to cause more than one person to walk into a lamppost and many more to talk to my chest as if it had a personality of its own. Running was not comfortable. As a teenager, I wore two swimsuits to avoid unwanted buoyancy. So, in my early thirties when I took up running, I wore two bras to avoid the bounce. It worked on that front but did nothing to divert the crass comments. But I continued running, and although plugging into music didn't drown out the running commentary on my chest ("Release the animals" was a memorable catcall), I perfected the art of the vacant stare past the culprits. Sports bra technology has improved over time and so the extra bra is no longer necessary. And although two pregnancies and age mean my chest has been unflatteringly described by my children as "long," continued running means it has actually shrunk a little and people are now more likely to talk directly to my face. Plus, through running (and now triathlons, too) I feel good about my body for the first time and no longer care what other people say or think about it. ■

2. I hate running.

Good. You would be a bit of a freak if you didn't. Everyone hates it until they have practiced it religiously for some time. Hating something shouldn't stop you from giving it a try. Hate and love are a hairbreadth away from each other—you know the cliché. So if you hate it (and with vitriol, like my husband), you are actually in a very strong position. You have passion, and once you take it up, you will love running at least as much as you once professed to hate it.

I REALIZED HOW much I had grown to love running on my wedding day. I'd been a bag of nerves the night before and barely slept. I knew that there was only one beauty remedy for it: I went running on the heath first thing in the morning. My sister came with me, and we both glowed all day. I like to think (although some of it was, of course, down to a beautiful dress and lovely hairdo) that my glow was certainly enhanced—as indeed was the experience of joy I felt that day—by that run.

3. I couldn't run in college. It's so boring.

No, being fat is boring and, worse, whining about being fat and doing nothing about it is even more boring. Don't you remember that most things were boring when you were at school? Being young, for example. Remember how much you wanted to be a grown-up and have a job? Couldn't have gotten that one more wrong now, could you? We are not in school anymore, so get over it. Immediately.

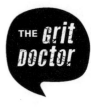

WILL SEE YOU NOW

Excuses, excuses. The Grit Doctor has heard them all. Take a number and keep reading— I'll get to all of you.

4. I don't have the time.

My personal pet peeve. Everyone has the same twenty-four hours a day. How do you think President Obama finds the time to go on his daily run? Or Michelle Obama—also fabulously fit and a multitasker extraordinaire? Do you think they conjure some extra time out of thin air? No. They have the same twenty-four hours as you, and I guarantee they have more to get done in any given day than you probably do in an entire week, and I mean a really busy week. Get over this one quickly. Get up earlier. Go to bed later. Or get organized and run to and/or from work. The latter option would most likely eat into the least amount of your time, if at all. Running is the least time-consuming of all sporting activities.

5. I need to do X first.

This is "I don't have the time" in disguise. It is the excuse that, on some unconscious level, is stopping you from attempting anything that challenges you. Accept that you can always tell yourself there is something else you need to do first. But this is just white noise. Ignore it.

6. It's raining; it's too cold; it's too dark; it's too windy.

Look at it this way: Neither the Super Bowl nor the New York City Marathon gets canceled because of the rain. Rain is no impediment whatsoever to a run. In many ways it is a bonus feature. There is nothing quite like the feeling you get if you stick your middle finger up to the worst of the elements and just run. The world rewards you for your efforts by making you look ten times rosier than you do after a run in less-arduous conditions and leaving you feeling like you could climb Everest. Dress appropriately and go for it. I promise you, when you have done this once you will never use the weather excuse again. You will wonder when you became the kind of person who gets up at six in the morning to go for a run—in the rain!

As for "it's too dark," don't be a scaredy-cat. Running in the dark is great, especially if you are feeling shy about how you might look as you venture out for the first time. The dark doesn't stop you from getting to the bar and back or from finding your way home from a shady nightclub in the wee hours. The only thing to remember is that you must take sensible precautions, most of which are common sense, but just to be on the safe side I have listed them in Appendix 1 (page 193).

7. I can't do it.

Yes. You. Can. (Repeat this to yourself over and over again in the style of President Obama for maximum effectiveness.) And in the next chapter, "The Six-Step Program," the Grit Doctor will show you how. You don't need a better body, and you don't need to get fitter first. You don't need more time. *You are ready for this exactly as you are.* You just need to read for a few more minutes and then get up off the sofa and out of your front door. It is as simple as that.

THE *grit doctor* SAYS

EITHER DO THIS thing or don't, but don't disempower yourself by making up excuses all the time. It is boring and makes you weak. Take a deep breath, shut out all the white noise in your head, and turn the page.

The Six-Step Program

Running makes you feel less deranged. . . .

There is a truly meditative quality to running that for me is a most cherished benefit. If I am anxious or afraid or just unbelievably stressed, nothing will cure me better than a good hour's running. Better still, if I am already feeling fantastic, going for a run can be almost hypnotizing. Everybody's experience is different, but all runners will know exactly what I am talking about. This morning Olly reported feeling incredibly peaceful and meditative during a run: "Sometimes my head becomes completely empty and I am able to think about nothing." This is a wonderful position to be in—freeing your brain up for anything or nothing.

So here we are! With luck, your sense of humor is still intact and you are feeling pumped about getting started. In six simple steps and over the course of eight weeks, I am going to teach you how to run. Follow the steps and **don't skip any**. You will need to use your common sense and be sensible about your limits.

Adapt this program to suit your own weight and fitness level without any fuss. The "breath test" (see page 54) is a great way to assess how well you are coping with your circuit and whether you are capable of upping it a notch. While on the subject of breathing—something so natural and instinctive—it is amazing how we can somehow lose the ability to do it effortlessly when learning to run, probably through anxiety and fear as much as through lack of fitness. Try practicing breathing slow, long, and deep breaths in through your nose and out through your mouth when you start your warm-up. This will help warm up the air and ensure that you use a bit more of your lung capacity, too. When you get better at it, focusing on your breathing during a run can be wonderfully meditative and a great distraction from all of the miles you may have left to run and from any niggling aches and pains in your body.

I am keenly aware that getting started may be the hardest part for you, and there is, of course, the all-consuming embarrassment factor. The buts, the ifs, the stuff that stops you from getting off your ass and out of the front door. You dig your sneakers out from your closet, you make promises to yourself and your other half, and you venture out once, only to give up, utterly humiliated that you were completely out of breath after ten minutes. This will not happen ever again if you follow the Grit Doctor's simple Six-Step Program. Because **anyone** of **any size** and **any age** can do this.

Fast Trackers, observe the six steps and get cracking. Slow Coaches, read the six steps and then follow the eight-week program in Chapter 4 (page 65).

STEP 1: You are on your own.

Drink a large glass of water. Wearing comfortable clothing and a pair of sneakers (don't buy new ones for the occasion—anything reasonably supportive will do at this stage), leave your front door and head out on foot for your nearest green space. If you have no access to a green space, walk through the streets near your house. Wherever possible, avoid concrete. **The aim of Step 1 is to walk out of your front door and create a loop that starts and ends at home. This ultimately will become your *running circuit.*** Wear a watch if you like so that you can time the whole outing, but there is no need to be overprecise about it. You want it to take roughly 1.5 hours door-to-door, which should work out to around 3 or 4 miles. Put in the time now and you will eventually be able to run your circuit in 45 minutes. Ideally the circuit should be relatively flat—with as little concrete as possible, to spare your joints. Somewhere you find interesting and pretty is a great bonus—but don't let an ugly neighborhood be your excuse not to run.

THE grit Doctor

WILL SEE YOU NOW

Q: But I live in a city. How can I stay away from concrete?

A: If there is no green space or local park available to you and you must run on concrete, in that case you really must invest in a pair of truly good running sneakers, as the concrete is very jarring for your knees and ankles. During the course of your circuit, whenever you spot a patch of green turf, track, or dirt trail, incorporate it into your run. Look online to find out where your nearest available green space is and practice your long weekend runs there. It always pays to escape the city once in a while, and you do need to do some of your runs on grass. It is actually harder because, unlike the concrete, your feet don't bounce straight off it. As a result, the grass is much better for improving fitness and stamina as well as putting less strain on those joints. It's win-win—so before you re-sign yourself to concrete running, explore your environment and do your research: You might find that at least part of your circuit can be run on a softer surface. If none of the above is possible because you live in the thick of a concrete jungle from which there is no escape except by air, invest in the best sneakers money can buy, always warm up carefully, and *grit out* running on the roads.

Your running circuit must, in fact, be a circuit—not several laps around the same park—just one continuous circuit home, ideally not covering the same ground twice. The reason for this is that laps can have the same effect as the treadmill: repetitious and boring, making your circuit seem unnecessarily hard. One continuous loop, on the other hand, gives you a sense of being on a journey with a beginning, middle, and end point, which the Grit Doctor believes is better for your running soul. Having said that, doing laps around a park beats running like a hamster on the treadmill hands down every time, so if it's a choice between those two, for God's sake go for the laps.

Walk the circuit at a comfortable pace. Unless you are completely out of shape you should be able to walk the circuit easily. If you are struggling, just slow down, but try not to stop. Speed up your walking pace if you feel comfortable. OK, well done. You've established a circuit, and you've walked it without stopping. This is a great beginning.

DO THIS FIRST circuit on your own. It is hard enough motivating yourself without the added burden of having to motivate someone else, too. A problem shared is, in this case, a problem doubled. At this stage friends will make everything much harder. Their broken plans, pathetic excuses, and negative, dispiriting chat will hold you back—"It's not working, let's join that Pilates class instead," "Ooh, let's have a milkshake, it won't kill us." It will. You can, of course, introduce newcomers to the practice, share with them what you have learned, and indeed run with them, but **only once you have "got it" yourself**. Step 1 is not the time to rope in a friend. This is about you, not anyone else.

STEP 2: Wax on, wax off.

Repeat Step 1 (page 50). In other words, walk your circuit again at a comfortable pace. Double-check with yourself that you really do like your circuit: that you enjoy the scenery, that it is long enough (minimum 1.5 hours walking door-to-door), that you are not intimidated by the other people you come across, that it isn't dangerous, that you won't get lost. Is there any way in which you would like to alter it, improve upon it, or lengthen it? If so, make the adjustments now. Are your clothes comfortable and supportive? Are your sneakers comfortable? You're not too hot or too cold? Good.

STEP 3: Do not run before you can walk.

Repeat Step 2 (above). Now walk it again tomorrow. And the next day. Walk it a bit faster each time or parts of it a bit faster each time. After a few days or weeks, depending on your starting weight and fitness level (which the Grit Doctor expects you to assess for yourself, using the easy method below), you should be building up your strength and walking more quickly and easily. You should be feeling confident about your route and relaxed because you are beginning to know it backward.

Don't be completely thrown by the idea of assessing your own fitness level. This does not mean you should get sidetracked by spending money on having your fitness assessed at a gym or getting your heart rate measured or any other nitpicky thing. **Just look in the mirror, preferably while naked, and have an honest conversation about where you are fitness-wise.** How many weeks or decades has it been since you last did any exercise? (And that *doesn't* mean a dash to the bus stop or tossing a ball around in the backyard.) What does your body actually look like? Can you see any muscles, or is everything buried under layers of flab? Be honest and realistic. **Even if you have done no exercise at all EVER and are extremely overweight, you can still do this program.**

THE *grit doctor* SAYS

IF YOU CAN pull yourself out of bed or off the sofa and make it to work or to go shopping, you are fit enough to start Step 1.

And remember there is **no running until walking your circuit has become second nature**; i.e., you can do it easily without becoming breathless and you feel totally ready—body and soul—to break into a slow jog. You will gain confidence about when you are ready to make the transition because your breathing will have improved considerably from your first outing, when the walk may have made you feel breathless. Plus, if you have been completely sedentary for some time, the weight probably will have started to come off just from the walking, which should be incredibly inspiring and help motivate you to continue.

If you are slim, don't be fooled into thinking you are necessarily any fitter. You can be very slim indeed and still incredibly unfit. For you skinnies who have done no exercise whatsoever, do the walk and see how you do.

THE BREATH TEST

The Breath Test is an excellent way to determine what you are capable of when on this running program. You should always be able to hold a conversation while walking fast and jogging slowly. If you cannot speak or say a sentence, you are overdoing it. On the other hand, if you can sing the national anthem, crank it up a gear.

STEP 4: Slow and steady wins the race.

OK, you are now ready to start running. Set out for your walk as you did in Steps 1, 2, and 3 (pages 50–53). After walking at a brisk pace for about ten minutes to warm up, allow yourself to break into the slowest sort of run you can imagine—a jog, really. There is something quite moving and humbling about the sounds of your pumping heart and rhythmic breath during a run, no matter how slow. You come to realize that you have this amazing body that is working perfectly. Get in touch with these sounds—the sounds of your body working—and learn to celebrate them. Give thanks that you are able to run—that you have these powerful legs and a full pair of lungs. Be proud that you are at last using them!

The difference between a fast walk and a very slow jog is this: When a fast walk turns into a slow jog, you bounce up and down a bit as your feet lift off the ground (no matter how slowly you jog, *you should always bounce*). The slow jog should follow on totally naturally from the pace of your fast walk. Break into this *very slow jog* and resist the urge to speed up. You will run out of steam too quickly. Go slow. Go slower. As slowly as is humanly possible. The aim is to go as slowly as you can for as long as you can without having to stop. As soon as you have to stop, it is time to walk, *not* to sit down, and certainly not to collapse on a park bench with your head between your knees, praying that you don't have a heart attack.

What I am saying here is that it's very important that you never stop moving. If you *have* to, it means that you have not been following the steps correctly and have overdone it, making it more likely that you will become injured. Once you are finished jogging (and, eventually, running) the entire circuit, you must always walk for 5 to 10 minutes afterward to cool down your muscles. Providing the circuit includes *at least* 40 to 45 minutes worth of attempted jogging, you can either build in a warm-up and cool-down as part of the circuit proper or add them to the start and finish. You are getting your body used to moving for longer periods of time, and the best way to ensure that you are doing this safely is to run for as long as you can at a pace that enables you to then walk the remainder of the circuit, thus building up your fitness levels at a realistic pace for you. Got it? Good.

THE *grit Doctor* SAYS

IF YOU BITE off more than you can chew, expect to feel sick.

Take a gentle "run-walk" through your circuit four or five times a week, and gradually build up the distance that you jog before you start walking again. The best way is to build on this from the same spot each day, trying to lengthen the distance you can jog before you walk the rest of it. Yes, you can break into another small trot later on after walking, but in order to measure your progress effectively, it's best to start from the same place and extend it, even if it's only by a few yards each day or 5 minutes each week.

If you are still in the "I don't have enough time" camp and are thinking this program is not for you because you can't do this four or five times a week: STOP THERE RIGHT NOW. Do it a couple of times a week until you are able to jog the whole circuit, and then squeeze in your extra runs when it is taking you less time. It will, of course, take you longer to improve. The magic only happens when you commit yourself to it three times a week *minimum*. There is something about three times a week or more that shifts the whole experience from being a huge effort into becoming more effortless. However, if it's twice or not at all, then I'll take twice if it is the *only* way to unglue you from the couch. When you are able to add in another run, do so immediately. Aim for at least three runs during the week, and then your weekend will feel like a proper weekend and your weekday runs are treated as "work." GET MOVING.

Ruth . . .

THIS PROGRAM WAS born when I moved back home for a year to live with my mother—then fifty-seven years old. I was thirty and eager to pay off the last of my student debt. (It had cost me sixty thousand dollars to become a trial attorney—insane career choice. Do not do it.) So my mother kindly took me in. Now I know how she feels about me. She loves me dearly and is very proud. But she also finds me a bit serious, a bit intense, and a bit of a food fascist, if you will. You see, Mom is a very relaxed and happy soul, so I know it was with a degree of trepidation that she accepted me back into the fold.

After I had done a ruthless spring cleaning of the kitchen—the fridge and all its contents, and all of the cabinets—we finally sat down to talk over a nice cup of tea. It was then that Mom revealed that she was ready to get fit and lose weight. She had enjoyed an active sports life right through her forties. She is also Catholic (this is a huge advantage, both for getting in touch with your inner bitch and for self-imposed grit of any kind). But at fifty-seven she had hit a wall. Without much energy, she was a bit down in the dumps about her weight and possibly a little bit lonely with Dad working abroad a lot of the time. I could barely contain my glee. What a wonderful project for me: to become my own mother's personal trainer and live-in dictator.

For Mom, the circuit was a lap around our local park, Virginia Water (or Vag Waters, as we call it). It is about a three-and-a-half-mile circuit. Mom was convinced she couldn't do this. That she was too fat, too old, too embarrassed. She had never run long distance before (although had enjoyed track and field in her youth). We started out just walking it. Marching, swinging our arms, chatting the whole way around. Then we started oh so very, very, slowly running—and I mean at a snail's pace—the first stretch of the circuit. Each day she extended the running stretch by a little bit, and before long (about two months later) she was able to run around the whole circuit very slowly, no problem. She was so pleased with herself.

This was five years ago. She still does that circuit but has added regular gym visits and swimming to her repertoire. She may still have the odd candy, but she also eats a lot more fish and green vegetables. She is no longer under any illusions as she is in touch with her inner bitch and has the voice of the Grit Doctor ringing in her ears whenever she digs into a scone. That hour around Vag Waters gave her back her confidence and sparkle and, more important, so much more energy to put into the rest of her life. Oh, yes, and she lost loads of weight. But you know what? After a while you forget about the weight loss. It becomes merely an incidental bonus and no longer your reason for running.

To: The Grit Doctor
From: Mom
Re: The Truth About Running

I stayed pretty fit after having four children until my early forties. But I hadn't done any exercise, really, for the last fifteen years and certainly not since going through menopause. I was missing it but honestly thought those days were gone for me.

When Ruth came home I was impressed by her committed approach to running and healthy eating, and noticed how much calmer and content she was after a run. Whenever she was in a bad mood, I would tell her to go running! I wished I could go with her sometimes but assumed I could never run as I was too old and too fat. Luckily Ruth had other ideas. She took me on as a sort of project, I think, determined that I could run, and I must say she was a very kind and persuasive coach.

I didn't get special shoes or a special bra, but we went to Virginia Waters and walked around it. It is about four miles, I think. It's a lovely walk by a lake and we chatted all the way. Ruth told me to walk briskly, swinging my arms as we went. After a few times just walking around she told me to jog with her for a bit, which I did. We did it so slowly it felt a bit silly but I still got tired quite quickly. She sensed this and told me to stop and walk the rest of the circuit. We probably only jogged for a minute that first time but she congratulated me at the end and I felt as though I had really achieved something. Each time we went I jogged a little farther. It was easy to improve each day because I would try and jog to a tree or to the bench just beyond the tree or to the swans just beyond that—always pushing myself the smallest amount farther.

One day I made it all the way to the halfway point around the lake. I couldn't believe I could get that far. I was thrilled and realized it wouldn't be long before I could go the whole way around. The first time I did I wasn't just pleased with myself, I was amazed. I told anyone who'd listen! I started doing it every day as I enjoyed it so much.

I always jogged very, very slow but when I finished I was hot and felt like I had done a lot of exercise. Ruth assured me I'd lose weight easily even at my age and it really did just fall off, despite my rather bad eating habits. And I was so much happier with myself. Getting up in the mornings for Mass, doing the food shopping and even the ironing—which I can't stand—seemed easier. I knew it was the running so I just stuck with it.

I must confess I hadn't run for a while around Vag Waters when Ruth told me about the book—I had been going to the gym instead and running on a treadmill—but since I read the book I've gotten right back into it, mainly because I am terrified of the Grit Doctor! ■

STEP 5: Keep waxing.

Repeat Step 4 (page 59) consistently. Stretch yourself little by little each time until you have completed the circuit by running all the way from start to finish (excluding the walking warm-up) without stopping. You will be so proud of yourself. By the time you do the entire circuit, you will be totally ready for it, having built up your stamina slowly and steadily at a rate suitable to your fitness level. You will have given yourself the best present ever. And it'll stay with you for the rest of your life. All you need to do is keep it up. Three times a week is the minimum, five times the optimum. The run should take you roughly 45 minutes door-to-door, and anything up to an hour is great.

To: The Grit Doctor
From: Olly
Re: Yes I Can

It was about six weeks after my first run that I finally completed my circuit without walking. It felt completely amazing. In the week leading up to it, I'd almost done it on a few occasions only to be foiled both times by the final steep slope up from the valley floor to the town square. A day or so later, I tried again, but this time, for whatever reason, I didn't even get close and ended up walking for the whole of the last fifteen minutes. It was incredibly frustrating. I had a day off after that, and it turned out to be a good idea, because it was the following day, fully refreshed, that I finally cracked it.

I remember the feeling of triumph that spread through my body on the uphill climb when I suddenly knew I was going to make it. I ended up sprinting the last few hundred yards like a madman, the blood pumping through my veins, my adrenaline through the roof, the *Rocky* theme playing in my head. It felt insanely good, and I couldn't wait to tell someone about it in unnecessary detail. Unfortunately for Ruth, there was no escape. ■

Finishing your circuit having run the whole way for the first time

GET OFF YOUR ASS AND RUN!   #gritdoctor

is probably not dissimilar to winning an Olympic gold medal. The feeling of joy and pride you will get from running the whole thing, knowing how when you started out you could barely manage five minutes, is unbeatable. But remember, none of it would have been possible without every single one of those incomplete runs that led up to it. *Every single one counts.* Every single time you put on your sneakers, brave the outdoors, and tackle your circuit is another step closer to gold. Chapter 4 (page 65) will help you get there.

A TIP FROM THE *grit Doctor*

DO NOT TRY to jazz things up by doing fancy warm-ups and stretches. You probably don't know how to do them properly anyway, and doing them incorrectly will make you look like a real loser. Walking briskly and swinging your arms is the perfect warm-up. Hold yourself up straight and pull your stomach and ass in. Try to maintain good posture at all times while running. Cool down in an identical fashion at the end of your run. Once you have been running regularly for at least six months, learning some good stretching and strengthening exercises and doing them regularly (especially before and after running) is a good investment against bursitis (inflammation) and other common injuries. See Appendix 2 (page 197) for some tips when this becomes relevant. No time wasting here please.

STEP 6: Get addicted.

Repeat Step 5 (page 59) three to five times per week, week after week, month after month, until you can't remember a time when you didn't do it. **Let it become who you are as opposed to something you do.** Get addicted. Treat yourself to a longer run once in a while. Go somewhere totally new. But only when you have really built up your confidence. Other runners will smile and nod knowingly in your direction. They, too, are in the club and may have been for many years. They are welcoming you in.

To: The Grit Doctor
From: Nicola
Re: Long Run, Short Run, Hot Run, Cold Run

Every day was a different run: short run, long run, fast run, slow run, jog and walk, sprint and jog, medium-distance slow, short-distance fast, cold run, warm run, hot run, good run, bad run. It all varied and I suppose that is when you truly come to love something, the moment you understand the subtleties that exist within an activity that to everyone on the outside looks exactly the same. ■

THE RUNNER'S REWARD

Now that you're a real runner, the time has come to indulge yourself in a trip to your nearest specialist running store. There are many fantastic specialist stores all across the United States, a few of which are listed in Appendix 2 (page 198). Be warned: The staff (undoubtedly all supremely fit runners) and the bewildering array of gear can be a tad intimidating for the novice. Have some running conversation and questions lined up ("I'm thinking of entering a 10K—any good ones you know of?," "Which sneakers are best for a bum knee?") before you enter with your head held high.

Once you are in, ignore all the clothes and supplies and focus on the shoes. They are different, very different, from normal sneakers, even those sneakers that claim to be running-specific. Do not fear the absurdly wide range of shoes on display. These shops work like magic. The assistant will tell you which pair you need and indeed which size you are. Believe it or not, you may not be the size you think for a properly fitting pair of running shoes. Explain to the salesperson that you want a pair of running shoes—and you can own up that it's your first pair—and before you know it you will be outside, running up and down under the watchful and highly trained eye of said assistant until she—not you—is satisfied that you have the right pair. This will set you back about a hundred bucks. But it's the best hundred bucks you'll ever spend. When you get home, put on your new shoes and take them out for a spin. Walking and running will feel so much better in these shoes. So different. So much easier. So much more comfortable. You will never ever want to run again in anything other than these perfect running shoes. Which is a very good thing because these shoes are your first line of defense against injury.

THE *grit doctor* SAYS

I AM NOT one for frivolities, but a good pair of running shoes is an absolute wardrobe essential once you are a practicing runner. Nonnegotiable.

To: The Grit Doctor
From: Olly
Re: Shoes!

Back in England for a few days and as a belated birthday pres-ent, Ruth took me along to Run and Become in Victoria to buy me my first pair of running shoes. It was time to cast aside the old tennis shoes I'd been using since my first French run and get into something new.

#gritdoctor   GET OFF YOUR ASS AND RUN!

Ruth had prepared me for the fact that this shop was a mecca of running, and she wasn't wrong. It had a lot of shoes in a very tight space. It also had a staff of indecently thin men and women who looked like they ran a marathon before breakfast. One of them proceeded to ask me an amazing number of questions about my feet and my running. She then selected about three pairs of sneakers and made me run up and down outside with them to see which one was the perfect fit. She wasn't just going to let me pick the first ones that felt OK. She wanted to find me the ones that would work in harmony with my running soul. And she did. ▪

Run with the Grit Doctor

Running makes you regular. . . .

If you suffer from constipation, running just might be the cure. Increasing your body's physical activity stimulates movement in your bowels, which is a very welcome side effect from catching the running bug. No fancy yogurt necessary.

T reat the six steps like the Ten Commandments—sacred and not to be argued or tampered with. For you Fast Trackers, the six steps alone may be all you need to get started. For those Slow Coaches among you, I have devised a day-by-day, eight-week program to literally walk you through those first steps into running a full circuit. Anyone, and I mean *anyone*, can do this—it is based on my mother's journey from walking to being able to run a 3.5-mile circuit. I have allocated two rest days per week, but you can take a maximum of three and a minimum of one, and you can vary this from week to week.

If you find it helpful to keep a journal of your progress, there is a running log at the back of this book designed to work in tandem with the eight-week program. Tear it out and stick it to your fridge if you think it will help you. But DO NOT be distracted by list-making, record-taking, and general time-wasting.

THE *grit Doctor* SAYS

INGRAIN THE SIX steps in your brain.

EIGHT-WEEK PROGRAM

WEEK 1

MONDAY

Read Step 1 (page 50), then plan yourself a suitable run that starts and ends at your front door (see Appendix 2, page 197, for mapping Web sites that can help with this). Remember, you will be walking this. I recommend a 3- to 4-mile circuit. So plan it and then walk it. Go on then, but don't waste too much time on the Internet. In fact, if you know this is a particular weakness of yours, don't map your run at all, just go outside, start walking, and use your imagination.

TUESDAY

Rest day.

WE INTERRUPT THIS CHAPTER WITH AN IMPORTANT MESSAGE FROM THE *Grit Doctor*

NO MATTER HOW tough your circuit was, or how thin you feel when you're finished, you never *ever* deserve two doughnuts afterward. Never stuff your face as a reward for your exertions. Get out of the bad habit of associating "naughty" foods with rewards for physical effort. NOTHING IN THIS LIFE BUYS YOU TWO DOUGHNUTS. Do *not* buy yourself two doughnuts unless you are diabetic and about to have a seizure.

While we are on the topic, no, you don't need a sports drink or a snack before a run, either. Your reward is the healthier, happier, slimmer you that regular running is treating you to.

GET OFF YOUR ASS AND RUN!   #gritdoctor

WEDNESDAY

Read Step 2 (page 52). Repeat Monday's walk.

THURSDAY

Read Step 3 (page 52). Repeat Wednesday's walk, but quicken your pace—swing those arms and march confidently around your circuit.

FRIDAY

Rest day.

A *grit doctor* REMINDER

REST DAYS ARE *not* reward days. Through committed running, you are rewarding yourself with a body that will love you for longer. Once you've nailed the running, your body just might stop craving the crap you used to put into it. That, or you'll develop enough grit to withstand the urge to pig out.

SATURDAY

Read Step 4 (page 54). Begin as on Thursday: **Walk the first 10 minutes**, then break into the **very slow jog** described in detail in Step 4 and sustain for **5 minutes**. Walk the remainder of the circuit.

THE *grit doctor* *WILL SEE YOU NOW*

Q: I can't seem to make it to five minutes no matter how slow I jog. What's wrong with me?

A: There is nothing wrong with you except that you are unfit. Five minutes jogging sounds a lot easier than it is. What you are doing is fine. Stick with whatever amount of time you can jog for now, and try to increase it by 30-second increments or by as much as you can manage each week. The program is a guide to which you should apply your own common sense and which you should tailor to your fitness level. Start using your own judgment. Listen to your body, stick with it, and SLOW DOWN.

SUNDAY

Repeat Saturday.

THE **Grit Doctor**'S GUIDE TO ACHES AND PAINS

IN ANY COMMITTED exercise routine there will be aches and pains and the odd twinge. The Grit Doctor expects you to tolerate these minor ailments and not to whine about them incessantly. Under the Grit Doctor's tutelage, you should build up your muscle tone gradually and shouldn't be in for any nasty surprises, but your muscles may feel tired to begin with, especially in the thighs and ass. Do not be put off by this. Should you even think of giving up, persevere and the side effects will reduce as your fitness level increases and your muscles firm up and adjust to being used properly.

Wear your pain with pride. This can actually be quite a pleasant feeling—the feeling of muscles having been put to use. Enjoy it. It is physical proof that you have pushed yourself outside your comfort zone: a badge of honor. Reflect with horror on how you have never felt anything in these places before and how inspiring it is that finally, after all this time, you are working those long-forgotten muscles. The odd stitch is no reason to worry, either. Drink more water (but don't guzzle down a gallon in one go just before setting out; instead, stay hydrated at all times). Refer to Appendix 1 (page 193) at the end of the book for advice on how to prevent serious injury and what to do if it happens.

You absolutely must not skip an exercise session because you have a stitch (an intense pain) in your side or because your muscles ache. This is simply your excuse-making machinery at work trying to thwart your attempts to change. Ignore it and soldier on.

WEEK 2

MONDAY
Rest.

TUESDAY
Repeat what you did last weekend—I'm referring to the walk/run, not the drinking binge.

WEDNESDAY
Repeat Tuesday, but extend the jogging part to **10 minutes** and *slow it down*. Walk the remainder of the circuit.

THURSDAY
Repeat Wednesday.

FRIDAY
Rest.

SATURDAY
Repeat Thursday.

SUNDAY
Repeat Saturday.

DISTINGUISHING BETWEEN GOOD PAIN AND BAD

Do not run with a temperature, if you are vomiting, or if you have diarrhea (this should be patently obvious), and be sure to wait until you are fully recovered before getting back into running, as your body needs all its energy reserves to stave off infection. If real illness strikes, you may need to go back a week or two in your running plan to rebuild your strength and stamina. Be sensible about it. If you have spent a month in intensive care recovering from malaria, be sure to take things really slowly and do a lot of walking before you attempt to run again. If, however, it was just a 24-hour bout of food poisoning, that shouldn't set you back more than a day or two of training—depending on how severe it was—so see how you feel, make sure you are properly hydrated before you set out, and take it slow.

THE *Grit Doctor* SAYS

A COMMON COLD is no excuse to put your feet up. If you've only got the sniffles, a run is not going to kill you. In fact, it might make you feel a lot better. But take it easy at first, and know your limits. Be responsible for your body and let common sense prevail.

WEEK 3

Start with a **10-minute walk** to warm up, followed by **15 minutes of incredibly slow jogging**, followed by walking for the remainder of the circuit without stopping. Take two nonconsecutive rest days of your choice.

UNLESS YOU'RE TAPERING down for a big race, you should never need to take two consecutive rest days! Nothing of any value in this life is gained without pain and sacrifice.

Ruth . . .

AS A GENERAL rule of thumb, I run one day and rest the next, which works out to three and four runs per week on alternate weeks. However, as soon as I take back-to-back rest days, two things happen: First, I need a much bigger push from within to haul my ass off the couch to go for my run on day three, and the run itself feels that much harder than it would have had I gone the previous day. Having said that, if I run on two consecutive days, it can go one of two ways: brilliantly easily or punishingly hard and more liable to set off a nagging pain in my knee. So I avoid doing that except when trying to extend myself or training for a race.

I am active, though—all the time—and I think this is also key to embrace as part of your new approach to fitness and health. Start getting into the habit of BEING an active person, someone who walks to places rather than drives, who walks (or runs) up the stairs instead of taking the elevator. It is no good just committing to your three weekly runs if you are spending all the rest of your time on the sofa, eating takeout. The idea is that the running gets you to be active and industrious in other ways, too, and gets you out of the bad habit of living a sedentary lifestyle.

#gritdoctor   GET OFF YOUR ASS AND RUN!

THE MOST IMPORTANT habit to cultivate is BEING A MORE ACTIVE PERSON. PERIOD.

WEEK 4

Ten-minute walk to warm up, followed by **20 minutes of jogging** (slow down the pace of the jog if necessary to sustain it for twenty minutes), followed by walking the remainder of the circuit without stopping. Two rest days, but not on consecutive days. Stick with the program.

THE *Grit Doctor*

WILL SEE YOU NOW

Q: I'm halfway through the program, but I'm going on vacation and I'm scared that I'm going to lose the last four weeks of training. What am I to do?

A: Circumstances should never dictate whether or not you go running. Quite the opposite in fact: the more difficult the circumstances of your life, the more important it is to keep running, because running will help you deal with whatever it is that you are going through. The rougher the week, the longer your weekend run ought to be.

The same approach applies to vacation, which can be a great time to squeeze in that sunrise beach run—the mother lode. By running on vacation, you can really enjoy your meals without worrying about gaining weight. It also gives you a chance to explore your new environment and really enhances the pleasure of being away from home. So if you are halfway through the program and off on vacation, just get out of your hotel room and set off as you would from home and create an appropriate circuit. Or, if it's a beach vacation, the length of the beach might provide an ideal run. It doesn't have to be perfect or precise, just so long as you are keeping it up so it is easy to pick up from where you left off as soon as you are home. This is one of the brilliant things about running: that you can do it whenever you like and wherever you find yourself, so geography is never an obstacle and most certainly should never be used as an excuse not to go.

WEEK 5

Ten-minute walk to warm up, followed by **20 minutes of jogging** (slowing down where necessary to avoid stopping altogether), followed by walking the remainder of the circuit without stopping. Two rest days as in previous weeks.

THE *grit Doctor* SAYS

IT DOES NOT matter how slowly you jog. Remember, the aim is to sustain your movement, either the jogging or the walking part, for the entire circuit without stopping.

WEEK 6

Ten-minute walk to warm up, followed by **30 minutes of very slow jogging**, followed by walking the remainder of the circuit without stopping. Two rest days.

WEEK 7

Ten-minute walk to warm up, followed by **35 minutes of very slow jogging**, followed by walking the remainder of the circuit—there may be almost nothing left! Two rest days.

WEEK 8

Ten-minute walk to warm up, followed by **45 minutes of very slow jogging**, followed by walking home if there is anything left of the circuit. If not, always cool down those muscles by walking a few hundred yards before you go back indoors—it's the ideal cool-down. Once you are able to complete the circuit, try to extend the jogging part to 45 minutes and then you are ready to start increasing your speed (should you so wish) as your fitness level improves. The sky is now the limit. Two rest days. **Read and observe Step 5 (page 59).**

WE INTERRUPT THIS CHAPTER WITH A MESSAGE FROM THE *Grit Doctor*

IF YOU HAVE made it this far through the book without actually running, now is the time to heed the advice of the title: GET OFF YOUR ASS AND RUN! Refer back to Step 1 and don't make me have to tell you twice.

WHAT NOW?

Read and observe Step 6 (page 61). Take time to congratulate yourself and really acknowledge your achievement. OK, that's enough. Consolidation is now key: absorbing your running routine

GET OFF YOUR ASS AND RUN!   #gritdoctor

into your weekly schedule and making it stick to you like glue. This bit is going to be easier than you think—you got over getting started, and that was the hardest part of all. Everything else is easy in comparison with that because you have done it gradually over time and slowly assimilated the regular practice of running into your very being. Once you are able to jog your circuit comfortably, of course you can run with a friend—of roughly the same level—if you find it motivating and enjoyable. And obviously do support and encourage anyone new to the program in any way you can. Telling them to GET OFF THEIR ASS AND RUN with a big smile on your face is always a good start.

A *Grit Doctor* ASIDE

THE GRIT DOCTOR maintains that the only way to "get it" initially is to go it alone. The eight-week program and the six steps are to be done by yourself while holding hands with your inner bitch *in order to properly establish your individual running pace without having to make allowances for others. Those eight weeks gritting it out* with only your inner bitch for company will really build your discipline of character. *It is meant to be hard.* Running with a friend and in a group is a treat that comes later on when and only when you are able to jog around your circuit comfortably.

Congratulations Fast Trackers and Slow Coaches alike: You are now 5K-race ready. When you have completed the eight-week program, if you are able to jog around your whole circuit without stopping, you are in the perfect condition to test out your race legs in a local 5K. There will be a huge number to choose from (consult Appendix 2, page 197, of the book).

Racing is incredibly exciting and nerve-racking, especially the first time. Don't be surprised if your body responds in kind and you find yourself stuck to the toilet the night before and the morning of your first race. The way to guard against your body reacting to these pre-race nerves is to practice by eating a tried-and-true supper the night before and a tried-and-true breakfast the morning of the race. Do this as many times as you like in the lead-up to race day—the same supper and the same breakfast at least 2 hours before setting out on a 5K run. You do not need to practice carb-loading or worry about tapering down before a 5K race. Which means: don't eat more or rest up in the weeks leading up to it.

Ruth . . .

GROUP RUNNING WAS an entirely alien concept to me until I ran a charity 5K with a group of women from work and my husband. It was a lot of fun to have scheduled group training sessions during lunchtime breaks and incredibly motivating, because I would be letting others down as well as myself in failing to show up, plus the running was so much easier—on account of all the gossiping with everyone the whole way around.

THE grit Doctor's DOS AND DON'TS
FOR THE MORNING OF YOUR 5K

DO eat breakfast at least 2 hours before the race and make sure you are fully hydrated.

DON'T guzzle water in the half hour leading up to the race as you may end up wetting yourself when the starting gun fires.

DO layer up. Races often begin in the morning, and there can be lots of standing around waiting beforehand, so wear layers that you can peel off easily.

DON'T race in new clothes and sneakers. Wear what you are used to running in comfortably.

DO get there early. There is nothing more stressful on race day than being late for registration. Pinning race numbers to T-shirts, waiting for the toilet—it all takes more time than you think.

DON'T carry anything to the start line: You won't need your phone, extra bananas, or drinks.

DO push yourself. Race-day adrenaline hopefully will propel you into a faster running time, so try hard to smash your personal best. And I want to hear all about it when you do @gritdoctor.

Besides that, no need to do anything fancy for race day. Stick to your routine and remember that nerves can be a good thing. Your inner bitch loves a hit of adrenaline.

As you continue to run, 5K or no 5K (yet), you will continue to notice all sorts of unexpected benefits—some instantly (higher energy levels, better sleep, improved mood), some later on (lowered cholesterol, more toned physique)—and you won't want to give them up.

If you have a great deal of weight to lose, then an even bigger "well done" to you because getting started was even harder due to the sheer physical burden of carrying that extra weight through the circuit. So you deserve a huge pat on the back. Keep it up. The weight will fall off. I promise you.

And no, you don't need your own special program if you are fat, although if you are morbidly obese (go to your doctor and ask), please seek medical advice before embarking on any kind of fitness program. I'm confident that any doctor would wholeheartedly endorse you strapping on a pair of sneakers and getting moving, albeit slowly. To be brutally frank, if you are morbidly obese, you won't be

#gritdoctor ● GET OFF YOUR ASS AND RUN!

able to manage anything more than moving very slowly anyway until some of the excess weight has shifted. You need to really focus on getting moving. NOW.

PUT YOUR FAITH IN A HIGHER POWER: THE RUNNING-STORE ASSISTANT

After a while, you'll start to notice that those shiny new sneakers you bought yourself are looking a bit shredded—usually after about 350 to 500 miles of running. (That sounds like a hell of a lot, but if you're running four miles four times a week, you could get through a pair of sneakers in around twenty-six weeks!) So it's time to head back to your local specialist running store. This is like your graduation. Armed with your battered pair of sneakers, head to the running store and go on about how you wore them out running around your circuit five times a week. You will immediately recognize the assistant as the same toned runner who sold you your first pair of proper sneakers (and is therefore something of a goddess); she, however, won't have a clue who you are as you are about half the size you were when you first went into the shop. Don't embarrass yourself here. She has been running for decades. Maintain an air of laid-back cool. You may think it's the greatest achievement in the world to have run in a 5K race, but this kind of person considers it commonplace. So you will return the shoes battered and worn to the assistant, who will inspect them and then choose you a new pair, most probably the very same shoe in an updated model. I love this process. That you don't get to choose, that the assistant decides. Like God. You put your trust in her. And she always gets it right.

THE GRIT DOCTOR does not approve of "runners" with special water bottles and straws coming out of book bags, with stuff attached to their arms and stopwatches and all that. And, incidentally, you don't need to drink throughout a 4-mile run provided you keep hydrated at all times during the day and drink plenty of water afterward. But as long as you don't let it distract from the thing itself—that's the run, in case you've forgotten—then anything goes. Buy and wear as much gear as you like, especially if you find it motivates you. If you must be plugged into an iPod, see the suggested running playlists in Appendix 4 (page 207), but be forewarned that you are in danger of not being able to hear that you are about to be overtaken.

Ruth . . .

I'VE BEEN RUNNING now for ten years and have had some wonderful (and some awful) experiences. Training for the London Marathon was, as you know, my first foray into running.

The race itself was extraordinary; over the course of it I seemed to experience every single emotion that I have ever felt: from complete despair to hope; anxiety, fear, and pain to incomparable joy. Totally weird and unexpected. I was moved to tears by a complete stranger who had terminal cancer but ran miles twenty-three to twenty-five by my side and prevented me from stopping. And I was moved to tears of another kind at the finish, this time frustration, by failing to overtake a guy with NO LEGS. Yep, I was beaten by a man with no legs.

But my greatest, or perhaps I should say most memorable, marathon experience was in New York. My old friend/nemesis Jane was running this one, too, and I was *determined* to beat her after the humiliation of my earlier defeat. I like to think I would have but for the fact that I had promised (practically by way of a blood oath) to look after my roommate, whom I had trained to run it and whose entire family had flown out to watch. Her father had made me swear not to leave her side throughout the run, and I was true to my word.

Jane had taken it upon herself to bring a mobile phone, a camera, and a banana to the start line. I looked at her and thought how silly she was to be so encumbered at the start of the marathon . . . and then she asked me to carry the banana for her. She then ripped the support from my sore knee and slid it onto her own leg, much to my roommate's escalating distress.

Why did I say yes to either of these requests, you may ask? Where was the Grit Doctor? Well, the truth is, I owed both girls—big time. For some reason we'd been really constipated since arriving in New York, and the night before the race I insisted we all take laxatives to sort ourselves out. I practically forced everyone to take double the dose to ensure it worked. This turned out to be a *very* big mistake. The next day we were all suffering from crippling tummy pains and had not gotten off the toilet all morning. I was entirely to blame, so lending a knee bandage and carrying a banana seemed a small penance in comparison.

My roommate wanted to go super slow, which was fair enough. Jane did not, so she abandoned us pretty early on—also fair enough. What was perhaps not fair enough was when my roommate decided to go so slowly she was, in fact, walking and I had to run backward and forward to keep myself going and be true to my promise not to abandon her. Five and a half hours later, we crossed the finish line, really running now and holding hands. It was very moving—I hope for both of us. The best thing though was the food we ate after the race. Her wonderful family took us to this fabulous restaurant where the portions were enormous (although, I am reliably told, paltry in comparison with the rest of America—note to self: must run marathon in another American state to sample portion size for myself), and we devoured about three cows' worth of ribs like scavenging dogs. Meat had never tasted so good.

Toward the end of the race, though, I kept thinking, *Next time, Ruth, you run for yourself. No people to look after and definitely no sharing of injury equipment. No carrying bananas, no artificial pace-setting by anyone else.* That was eight years ago, and sadly there has not yet been a next time. I really want to run a marathon with my sister or my brother or my mom, or perhaps all four of us together, in a country we have not yet visited.

I do have some wonderful memories, though, of running with my sister, particularly from when we went to Kenya together on vacation. All we needed to get us to run was the Grit Doctor, who came along in our suitcases. She leaped out the first morning at about five AM, beckoning us down to the beach to go running. We had talked a lot about running on this vacation, so it was in an almost holy silence that we put on swimwear and T-shirts and tiptoed outside to make the short three-minute walk to the beach, where we started to run.

This was a six-mile stretch of coastline, littered with hazards: Some parts felt quite dangerous, areas where the sand was less smooth and bits where we were followed by slightly mangy-looking dogs. But by day three we had our run nailed. The best thing about it was seeing all these young Kenyan men and children at the crack of dawn, training on the beach, doing sit-ups and push-ups, sprints, interval training, and long-distance runs, and without fail, one or two would join our run. When we got to the end, back to the resort, morning had broken and we dove into the sea in total ecstasy before tucking into an enormous breakfast buffet. My sister still teases me about how un-vacationish our vacation was on account of all the running (and reading) that took place, but I know she loved it. Wherever she goes, she is sure to run—it is the best way to make friends with a new environment and feel as relaxed and happy as you ought to on vacation. It also leads to guilt-free eating, of course! I must say that we both came back from that trip with a real glow.

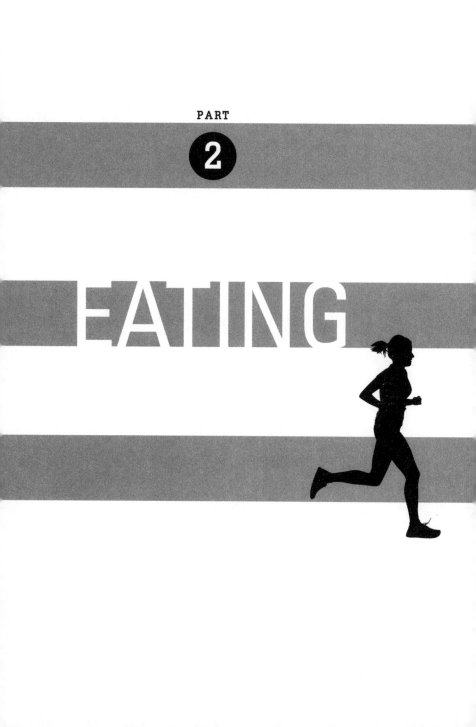

EATING

5

Run Yourself Thin

Running helps you score. . . .

Before I got married, if I had a date on a Friday or Saturday night, I always made sure that I went on a run beforehand. The run would calm my nerves and ensure I was relaxed, chatty, and genuinely happy, and I also knew I would be looking my absolute best.

You will be so pleased with yourself for fitting in a run, and that translates into looking good—let alone the very real physiological transformation of your glowing complexion. You won't have that horrid loss of appetite that ruins many a good date, either. Your date will find you way more attractive if you order the burger and chips and actually manage to eat them. Plus, you won't need to down ten gin and tonics beforehand for courage; the run will give you all the courage you need. You will glow and you will enjoy yourself.

YOU NEED TO complete Part 1 of this book before you can go on to make any of the changes in Part 2. Running and the practice of running are what your diet is all about. After all, sweat is fat crying and hopefully you will have produced oceans of tears already. By all means read on now, but ensure that you have completed the Six-Step Program in Chapter 3 (page 47) and are committed to running regularly before you even think about changing your eating habits. Ignore the Grit Doctor at your peril.

I have a real problem with the word *diet*. It is invariably used to mean weight loss. This is not what the word *diet* really means—in fact, the *Oxford English Dictionary*'s primary definition is "way of living or thinking," which seems to me to be a much healthier interpretation of the word. But because you almost certainly associate *diet* with punishing weight-loss regimes, we're going to try to use a different word in its place wherever possible: FOOD. Because you are not going on a diet as you know it. You are running regularly and losing weight. What you now need is the right fuel to accommodate your new lifestyle and burgeoning appetite. The great bonus is that you will want all this food anyway because, if you've been running, your body will be crying out for it. In short, the hard part was getting you running. The food part is EASY.

#gritdoctor

GET OFF YOUR ASS AND RUN!

FAT VERSUS THIN

Your past relationship with food and your current body shape will influence how you read this next section and what you take from it.

If you are **thin** and have no desire to change your weight at all, you still need to read Part 2 because it's possible you're not eating enough and you may not be eating the right sort of food to fuel your running.

If you are **overweight**, you will lose weight quite effortlessly through running. But you probably have some bad eating habits that you should change in order to keep yourself fit, healthy, and, crucially, able to continue running regularly.

If you are **very overweight** or even morbidly obese and are not losing enough weight through running and are struggling to run because of the excess weight, **READ THIS SECTION VERY CAREFULLY INDEED** and consult your doctor.

GRAVE AND WEIGHTY MATTERS

So how do you figure out the truth about your own body shape? Well, you've already done the naked mirror assessment, and hopefully the Grit Doctor has forced you to confront your wobbly bits. But for the purposes of this next section, I recommend you weigh yourself *just once*. It is extraordinary how many people lie about their weight, as much to themselves as to others. Women who say "I'm about 120" when they are frankly closer to 150 do other women a serious disservice. It's your real weight we want, please, *not* your fantasy weight. You are not the weight you were as a teenager when you last got on the scales at a compulsory school medical exam. Just because you can still *squeeze* into the same pair of jeans you wore ten years ago does not mean that you are the same weight.

Go to your local pharmacy, one that has a set of electronic scales that can print out your weight and Body Mass Index (BMI). You can even work it out for yourself using an online calculator (try cdc.gov /healthyweight/assessing/bmi/adult_bmi/english_bmi_calculator /bmi_calculator.html) or for added grit factor seek a professional medical opinion. When you've got the results, DO NOT try to cheer yourself up. Acknowledge the awful fat truth—it is extremely useful fuel for your running engine and should have you back outside conquering the streets before the day is out. (And be thankful that the weighing-in part of this book came *after* you started running, not before. Just think what the number could have been. . . .)

THE *grit Doctor*'s ORDERS

DO NOT BUY yourself a set of scales. You will only waste valuable running time obsessively weighing yourself—and stepping on and off the scales *doesn't* count as exercise.

TARGET WEIGHT

Now that you know your real weight, identify your target weight. This is where you put away the picture of Victoria Beckham you used to spur you on in your early runs. I'm talking about the ideal *healthy* weight for your age and height. *Do not create an unhealthy target weight inappropriate to your age and height.* DO NOT GUESS. Use the online calculator or ask your doctor. And always bear in mind, especially when you feel overwhelmed by how many pounds you still have to lose, that 90 percent of the work is already done. I kid you not. Because 90 percent of your "diet" is continuing to run three to five times every week. And each week, the pounds will continue to fall away.

CAN'T SEEM TO LOSE THAT FAT ASS?

Most runners tend to be fairly healthy eaters because once you get fitter you naturally care more about what you put into your body; plus, you need the right sort of fuel to run efficiently. Because you are happier, you will also be less inclined to eat away negative feelings, a vicious cycle many people get caught up in. Six months into your running program, without any dramatic changes to your diet, and I believe you will be closing in on your target weight. How close you are depends on where you started, but if you don't seem to be losing as much weight as I promised you, it is most likely because you are eating too much of the wrong foods.

This section on food is going to be short. Dieting and diets are extremely boring topics. Remember that the beauty of running is that not only does it make adopting new and better practices in other areas of your life so much easier, but *it*, the run, also will act as your "diet."

I hope that you are already at the point where you *want* to eat more healthily. It is a weird side effect of running. And so when this does happen, the Grit Doctor wants to be there to help you make good food choices. That is what this section is about. IT IS NOT ABOUT DIETING. THERE IS NO DIET. YOUR RUN IS YOUR DIET.

Once you get into your running routine and experience a surge in appetite, it pays to stock up on the right foods and acquire some good habits in order to accommodate your raging hunger. If you are relatively healthy anyway, with no nasty eating habits, then you genuinely do not need to change a thing. Just stick to the **two golden rules** that follow, and continue running. *The weight will fall off.* You can really enjoy your food and not worry about making any drastic changes. However, if you are regularly eating foods on the Seven Deadly Sins list (page 109), then you are filling yourself up with junk and useless calories. This will make running more difficult and your weight loss less dramatic. You need to be healthy to be a practicing runner, and you need good fuel for your body. But you don't ever need to skimp on portion sizes or deprive yourself of a treat (or, indeed, the odd blow-out, indulgent calorie-fest) because it is running that is keeping you thin, not your food choices.

If you feel that you are really fat and need to make some drastic changes to the way you eat, then I suggest you follow the ideas in this section very carefully. You probably know what it is that you need to stop eating and you know what you should be eating instead, but so far you have chosen to ignore the obvious. However, there is good news. You have transformed yourself into a runner and that brings with it an *automatic shift* in your attitude to your body and what you choose to put into it. Capitalize on this change of attitude, and take advantage of the increased motivation you have developed through running to tackle your food issues.

This is why it is so important to master the running first. It gives you the vital energy and motivation to assure your success on the food front. Whether you have the odd bit of tweaking to do or you need to radically overhaul your eating patterns, you will be able to confront this issue much more effectively as a runner. So what follows in the next five chapters are the **two golden rules** and some tips to take on board, which will be nothing short of a pleasure for you, a committed runner in touch with her inner bitch, to now embrace.

THE grit doctor

WILL SEE YOU NOW

Q: But . . . I smoke half a pack a day and I get winded quite easily. I am 35 years old and have not done any serious exercise since being on the high school baseball team. Does this mean I can't take on the six steps and the eight-week program?

A: Absolutely not. Smoking (just like being fat) is no barrier to embracing the six steps. The good news is that once you have that circuit nailed you are going to come to hate those cancer sticks. You will feel firsthand how they are limiting you and holding you back from realizing your full potential. You will want to enjoy the full capacity of your lungs so you can take on a hill without feeling as though you are about to have an asthma attack— and you are going to want to quit. Running is a big step toward giving up smoking. It will also help stave off any potential weight gain when you do give it up because the running hopefully will burn off that extra food you may crave.

The program may be harder for you—*suck it up*. You may start coughing up a lot of gunk from those smoke-addled lungs— *be horrified*. And then one day you are going to wake up and want to run farther faster, and the only thing stopping you is your smoking habit. It boils down to a simple choice. The *inner grit* you will have acquired through the eight-week program, the extra fitness, the awareness of your body, and an increased desire to cherish it all will help you make the right choice. Don't take a moment while this all sinks in to light up a cigarette. Lace up your sneakers, turn to page 50, and BEGIN STEP 1 NOW.

The Two Golden Rules

Running buys you time. . . .

If I have something I really don't want to do (usually work-related), I know that if I go on a run first, I will be able to complete it more quickly and do a better job. Even though the run itself eats forty-five minutes into my evening, the work will be finished earlier than if I didn't go on the run. It is a very strange paradox. A run is an investment in time. So never think of it as time out but rather as time multiplied.

Rule #1

DRINK MORE WATER.

Rule #2

EAT
LESS
CRAP.

Dieting Delusions

Running gives you great legs. . . .

Not only is it the ultimate calorie burner for all-around body improvement, it is the only exercise I have found that really tones those parts of a woman that are especially prone to sag— in particular, the thighs and butt. I'm convinced it banishes cellulite. Having good legs enables you to wear all sorts of clothes that you otherwise might shy away from post-thirty, like shorts and miniskirts, and to look really good in them. And who doesn't want great legs?

Running is a brilliantly effective way of getting you into the habit of caring for your body: caring about what you put into it just as much as what you can get out of it, and realizing what your body is capable of when you begin to exercise some serious discipline over it. None of it is easy, though, so don't expect to be able to completely override all of your bad eating habits overnight. Some of them are deeply embedded and will require *MUCHO* grit to banish for good. Some habits come complete with excuses that prevent us from taking those essential first steps toward transformation.

Some of these "dieting delusions" I have listed here, but others will be unique to you. If you are overweight and keep citing a "reason" for it that you think makes you different from everyone else, ADD IT TO THIS LIST. The more compelling the reason to you, the more ridiculous it will invariably be in the eyes of the Grit Doctor. Nine times out of ten, it is either an excuse or a delusion that you need to obliterate in order to even begin to grapple with your food issues.

Always bear in mind that a good habit (once made) is just as easy to maintain as a bad one. Repetition is the fuel of habit-making. Wax on, wax off.

"I'LL START THE DIET TOMORROW."

This is the main reason why you are unable to give up being fat. It is not about starting a diet. It is about changing some bad habits.

And *right now* is the only time you've got. Pour yourself a glass of water, put a potato in the oven, and make that the beginning. Next, throw out all your fat-laden foods and treats. Exorcise your cabinets and fridge, and give them a good spring cleaning. Go to the supermarket, on foot if you can, and stock up on all things good for you. Take a peek at the list of good foods in Chapter 9 (page 113) for inspiration. Do this now and it will be a very strong beginning—and as we already know, *getting started is the hardest part of all.*

It is really important to lose the whole concept of dieting in your quest for a fitter, healthier, and slimmer you. I cannot reiterate enough the importance of GIVING UP DIETS. And while you're at it, give up "starting stuff tomorrow." Start it now. Whatever it is. DO IT NOW.

THE grit doctor SAYS

DIETING IS A dirty word. Eating should never be about slavishly following a diet. It is about changing habits, shifting attitudes, and taking responsibility for your body.

"I'LL START EXERCISING ONCE MY DIET WORKS."

Wrong. As we've already discussed, it's *the other way around.* This bears repeating because it's a really dangerous concept that needs to be challenged. *You need to get running first in order to start feeling good about yourself.* It's only when this begins to happen that you will want to eat more healthily. Any dietary changes you need to make will actually be far easier to embrace once you are a committed runner, because a happier, fitter you is in a much stronger position to change. In fact, healthier eating habits will come quite naturally once you have established a good running routine. Move more, eat less (crap).

THE *grit Doctor* SAYS

DON'T GIVE UP. There is a permanent escape route from a life spent trapped in a fat body, and running will help you find it.

"I'M BIG-BONED."

Really? Are you? If you genuinely think this might be the case, get a professional opinion. Go to the doctor, get weighed, and ask if you are overweight. You may be big-boned, but you may also be fat. Being big-boned is no excuse for being overweight. Chances are you are kidding yourself.

"I DON'T LIKE VEGETABLES AND SALAD."

You clearly didn't get scolded enough as a child for not eating your greens. This whole thing is going to be a lot harder for you. Spoiled brats can be very resistant to grit. But imagine how much you would impress others (others being people *other* than fellow spoiled brats) if you were able somehow to change something about yourself? That you are reading this book is a very impressive beginning.

"I DON'T LIKE WATER."

I am not asking you to *like* water. I am telling you to drink it. There is a distinction between the two. I don't think to myself, "Ooh, yum, I'd love nothing more right now than another glass of tap water!" Nobody does. Water is essential fuel for all your bodily functions, and upping your intake is fundamental to running safely and to the success of any long-term "healthier you" plan. Herbal teas are fine, and carbonated water is a delicious treat: with fresh mint, or cucumber and elderflower, or just a squeeze of lemon or lime—deliciously refreshing.

THE *grit Doctor* SAYS

THE GRIT DOCTOR is depressed that something as simple as drinking more water is such a barrier for so many people. Really, what's wrong with you people? In place of water you drink fizzy drinks and endless cups of tea and coffee. Not only are these drinks full of useless calories, but most of them also act as a diuretic, so they *de*hydrate rather than *re*hydrate, making you thirsty, tired, and lacking in energy. For the love of God, drink more water.

"I HAVE A REALLY SLOW METABOLISM."

Bullshit. You are overweight because you eat too much of the wrong food.

The Grit Doctor's Plan for Permanent Weight Loss

Running gets boring work done. . . .

No, not literally. But my God it helps. Ironing. Doing the dishes. Dusting. Vacuuming. Grocery shopping. Tax returns. Running makes all those deadly boring daily tasks easier to do. My theory is that because of the happy hormones that running stimulates, you become much better at "getting on with life" without so much resistance and complaint. Everything is easier to bear after a run. Consequently, you get everything done much more quickly and efficiently.

THE SEVEN DEADLY SINS

1. **Soda** is crack cocaine without the weight-loss benefits. It has no place in the fridge. Not even the diet kind, which is also filthy and disgusting and makes your breath stink. Do everyone a favor and give it up. The only fizzy drink you should ever consider consuming is seltzer. And champagne. And don't try to fool yourself into thinking sweetened iced tea or fruit juices are any better.

2. **Candy** is for children and has no place in an adult's life. Grow up. Give it up.

3. No more **snacking** . . .

4. This includes **chips, cake, and cookies.**

5. **Pastry** is dangerous. Delicious and dangerous. I feel strongly about this, partly because it seemed to be an essential part of my daily pregnancy needs, and wow, did it pile on the pounds. Remind yourself that pastry is basically butter: totally delicious, flaky buttery heaven. Anything that tastes that good is going to be bad for you. If you do cave in to temptation and eat it, be sure to enjoy a punishing run that day. This should help to prevent a relapse.

6. **Fast food** and . . .

7. **Takeout**, the Grit Doctor's bête noire. Not only is takeout food incredibly fattening and nutritionally deficient, it encourages the sort of couch-potato living that you are trying to reject.

IF YOU ARE consuming any of the aforementioned sin foods as part of your daily diet, this is the reason you are not losing as much weight as you would expect from running alone. Frankly, as an adult, you should be ashamed of yourself if you are still buying candy and soda on a weekly basis. Stop it now.

THE GRIT DOCTOR'S ORDERS

Practice mindful eating. In other words, before you shove anything down your piehole, ask yourself these three questions:

1. **Why am I eating this?** (To which the only acceptable answer is: "Because it is mealtime and I am hungry.")
2. **Is this good for me, or is it just junk keeping me trapped inside this overweight body?**
3. **What would the Grit Doctor say if she saw me now?**

And always follow the Grit Doctor's Orders:

- Eat only three meals a day and eat them *at mealtimes.*
- Eat your evening meal *early.*
- Eat slowly and chew thoroughly. As with running, *slow down.*
- Eat *smaller portions*, especially of the bad stuff.
- Load up your plate with *vegetables*, preferably green ones. Ideally, half of your plate at mealtimes should be made up of vegetables.

- Use *less oil and fat* in cooking, and spread butter thinly. Be really anal about this.
- *Cut down on desserts*. They are not a daily staple but a treat. Fresh fruit and natural yogurt are exceptions to this rule.

AND, LEST YOU FORGET:

- Make *running* three to five times a week a habit. Get it into your head that your run is your diet.
- Drink water. *Drink more water.*

THE *grit doctor* SAYS

THERE IS SO much nonsense out there about diets and weight loss that it is very easy to get completely overloaded with advice (which is often useless) and embroiled in overly complicated food regimens. Do not get sidetracked by all the dieting information out there. It is all a complete waste of time and commits you to a very boring lifestyle. You can be slim and eat normally if you run at least three times a week.

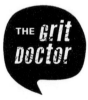

THE *grit doctor*

WILL SEE YOU NOW

Q: But . . . I have been running regularly for three months now, and the weight came off to begin with but seems to have plateaued. I was very focused for our son's wedding, which was two weeks ago, and since then I must admit to being a bit hit-and-miss with the eating. Do I need to increase my runs to start losing weight again? I am running three times a week for 45 minutes. I still have a lot of weight to lose. My BMI is 35.

GET OFF YOUR ASS AND RUN!

A: The initial weight loss was no doubt entirely down to introducing exercise in a big way into your previously sedentary lifestyle. It was a welcome shock to your body, which responded by burning off some of the excess fat. What has happened is that your body has now recalibrated itself to account for the exercise, which has clearly not been accompanied by a shift in your eating habits. At a BMI of 35, you must address your eating habits.

It can help in the early stages to have a specific occasion in mind (your son's wedding) to work toward to help keep you focused and motivated on your runs and away from the cake. However, in the long term, this approach is bound to fail. If you're trying to lose weight for a specific event, you have slipped into "diet" mode. FATAL. You need to start seeing losing weight and getting fit as VITAL to your health and well-being. This isn't about looking good for your son's wedding; it's about living long enough to see your grandson get married. Use the gritty reality to create a shift in attitude toward food and exercise *for the rest of your life*.

Keep running. You can mix up your thrice-weekly runs a bit, take on a small hill (very slowly), or speed up for short portions of your circuit if you feel able. There are loads more benefits coming your way in time if you stick with it, including a healthier attitude toward food. Why not enter a race in 4 to 6 months' time and make that a goal, one that will have the impact of keeping you running and hopefully eating better foods to fuel those training runs? Give up eating junk. TODAY.

9

Good Foods

Running gives you a flat stomach. . . .

During a run, think about your posture and use the run to improve it. Regular running will make you proud of your stomach by making the flab disappear and toning up the underlying muscles at the same time quite effortlessly.

For extra midriff tone, try to get into the habit of running while tensing your stomach muscles. Sound deranged? It is. Imagine your back in the position it would be in if you were doing a sit-up correctly—the small of your back pressed into the floor, tummy held in, tail tucked under—and try to re-create this posture while running. It is not easy, and I often forget to do it myself, but at the very least, get into the habit of holding your stomach in and lengthening your torso while you run.

f you want to make progress, your body needs good, honest fuel. What follows are just some examples of good foods that you should introduce in a big way into your diet. It is by no means an exhaustive list. If you are at your target weight, you are hopefully already eating the right foods. If you are the wrong weight, sit up and pay close attention.

- **Pasta and bread.** Yes, those very foods that are often the ones most diets tell you to give up should be eaten by the boatload. HOO-bloody-RAY. Except for the wheat- or gluten-intolerant runner, **pasta and bread are absolute staples**. Eat them without a trace of guilt. The butter and sauces and jams and cheese that we slather on top of them are what make them fattening, not the pasta and bread themselves. Obviously whole wheat bread is better than white. But if you must use butter, spread it *really* thinly. At all times. Scrape off any excess bits. Every little bit counts. It is, after all, pure fat.
- **Potatoes.** Another thing they say you should give up on a "diet." I beg to differ. A baked potato is another perfect food for the committed runner. Just throw one into the oven before you set out on a long run to devour upon your return, all crispy on the outside and creamily fluffy on the inside. Mashed up with some cheese, butter (remember the rules), and fresh herbs, they can't be beaten.

- **Raw vegetables.** As already stated, you should make green your favorite color. Remember that, for most vegetables, the closer they are to raw, the better. Steam or lightly boil them to retain their goodness. Keep raw vegetables in the fridge for snacking—carrots, cucumber, peppers, etc. You will need plenty of healthy snacks available to accommodate your increased appetite. If vegetables alone aren't enough to fill you up, skip the high-fat vegetable dips and choose tzatziki instead.
- **Lean red meat.** Perfect for replenishing iron stores and much-needed protein. For vegetarians, cheese, yogurt, and eggs are the obvious staples, and for vegans, tofu, beans, and almonds are good sources.
- **Fish.** Obviously. Not only fresh fish, which can be expensive, but canned sardines, mackerel, or tuna on whole wheat toast or a bagel are fantastically nutritious.
- **Whole-grain cereals and oatmeal.** Ideal fuel for running. Eat with skim or nonfat milk. Or water if you are in the mood for self-flagellation.
- **Chocolate (especially dark)** can be eaten *in moderation*. It is not normal to eat a bar of chocolate every day as part of your lunch, but chocolate is a great energy-boosting treat before, after, or indeed during a run (just ask women's marathon world-record holder Paula Radcliffe).
- **Fresh fruit and yogurt.** Stock up on these for snack attacks.
- **Dried fruit and nuts, whole wheat crackers, rye crispbreads, and the like.** Ditto.

When you are running regularly and eating healthful foods like these, you'll be less inclined to overeat and your body will use the food as fuel, not store it as fat. That means that—within reason—you can basically eat all of these foods as much as you like

THE *grit doctor* SAYS

TRYING TO FIND low-fat versions of your favorite junk foods (low-fat potato chips, low-fat chocolate bars, low-fat or sugar-free cookies) is *fatal.* It only serves to keep you trapped in your bad habits, such as having a bag of potato chips with your lunch. It is still a bad habit, even when disguised as a low-calorie/low-fat/low-sugar alternative, which is more often than not packed full of junk ingredients. The idea is to get out of the old bad habits and into forming new good ones. Raw vegetables, fruit, and yogurt are what you want to train your brain to be craving with lunch, not a bag of chips.

The Grit Doctor Kitchen Control

Running helps you sleep. . . .

This was a massive and unexpected bonus for me when I took up running. I never got so good at sleeping as I did after I started running. I experienced once again the sort of teenage and pre-teenage sleeping scenarios that I had long since forgotten: falling straight to sleep when my head hit the pillow—and not only that but into a deep and satisfying sleep. Heaven. None of that staying awake for ages with thoughts and anxieties racing through my head. A good run on any given day almost certainly guarantees a good night's sleep thereafter.

am not a chef and this is not a cookbook, but there are a couple of basic staples that every runner should have in their culinary arsenal. Quick, nutritious, and *tasty*, they are also brilliant for any of you who suffer those guilt-ridden God-I-really-ought-to-cook-my-children-something-from-scratch-like-Jamie-Oliver-does moments. The key is to learn a few simple bases you can cook without even having to think about the ingredients, quantities, or method. Then you can get as creative as you want to, jazzing them up as the mood takes you. It's a bit like mastering your basic running route before you start going off course.

THE *Grit Doctor* SAYS

TAKE CONTROL OF your eating habits. Start cooking your meals from scratch using fresh ingredients. No more slavishly following the latest diet fad or hot new chef. You are in control now, and you need to start thinking for yourself.

Before you object with the "I don't have the time" excuse or "I can't afford it," this is fast and economical cooking at its best. You need to get back in touch with what it is that you are putting into your body and begin to exercise the same discipline over your kitchen as you are exercising over your running.

DON'T GO OVERBOARD in following any eating regimen. The rules are there to be broken every once in a while, provided you are running at least three to five times a week. Indeed, you can break the rules regularly *once you have reached your target weight*. The Grit Doctor wants you to take responsibility for your weight and your body without becoming some sort of birdseed-munching health freak.

PASTA

As we've already discovered, pasta is the runner's friend. But sauce and cheese are not. The key with any type of pasta sauce is "less is more"— less sauce means you can eat more pasta. Crushed raw garlic and thinly sliced chile peppers stirred through piping hot spaghetti al dente with a drizzle (not a gallon) of olive oil, chopped herbs (parsley or basil always work), seasoning, and Parmesan (grated on the thinnest part of the grater so you use the least amount of cheese) is a delicious and filling meal, not to mention incredibly quick and easy to prepare.

To this great base you can add any number of other ingredients. Finely chop shallots or onion, sweat them in a pan with a smidgen of oil, and then chuck in some veggies. Frozen edamame are a great freezer staple that I add to loads of dishes, but you can also try cherry tomatoes, broccoli florets, or peppers, to name but a few. Add strips of cooked meat if that's your thing—ham, chicken (leftovers are great for this). Crumbled feta cheese or mozzarella (in smallish quantities) can be stirred through instead of Parmesan.

Or try a classic tomato sauce—there are loads of easy recipes out there (avoid any that say you should remove the tomato skin— who has that kind of time?). If you make loads and freeze it, you'll always have a meal on standby. Again, you can spice the recipe up with roasted vegetables or meats.

Before long you will have developed your very own repertoire of pasta supper recipes—fuss-free and delicious.

SOUPS

Again, get the base right and you can create and develop your own recipes. Sweat a chopped onion with finely diced celery (garlic is optional) in a little oil and butter (listen for the voice of the Grit Doctor when you're adding in fats). Then add your vegetables, cut roughly into bite-size chunks, and sweat until softened. Next add chicken or vegetable stock (fresh is best, but a cube will do) and simmer very gently for a maximum of 20 minutes. Don't boil it to death or you will lose all the goodness from the veggies. Mix with an immersion blender or in a Vitamix, or mash with your potato masher if you don't have the appliances or just love added grit factor. Continue until you have the consistency you like. Add more boiling water to thin if necessary. Parsley is a great herb for flavoring soups at the end, and it's extremely good for you, being high in calcium and vitamin C.

Make a big batch, as your soup will keep in the fridge for up to 3 days and provide you with an ideal meal after a good run. You can also freeze batches in individual portions to help organize your eating.

THE *Grit Doctor* SAYS

IF YOU HAVE a long-standing weight problem and are trying to lose weight, it is a good idea to plan your meals at the beginning of the day or even for the entire week, leaving no room for later excuses or possible meltdowns. This is why it helps to have frozen batches of soup and other healthy meals ready to reheat. Keep mealtimes and choices simple and uncomplicated.

STIR-FRY

Get a wok. The stir-fry is another Grit Doctor staple. It is unbelievably quick to prepare, and the method of cooking ensures the vegetables retain all their goodness.

Use the tiniest amount of oil and heat for a minute on a very high heat. Then throw in a chopped onion, finely chopped chile peppers, garlic, and ginger, and then add prawns or diced chicken, beef, or pork (as lean as you can) and stir-fry for a good 5 minutes. Then throw in some raw vegetables for a couple of minutes. Keep stirring. Add some cooked noodles or rice at the last minute and a splash of soy sauce if that's your thing. *Voilà*: instant, healthy goodness.

THE *Grit Doctor* SAYS

STEER CLEAR OF all ready-made sauces—they are invariably full of junk and hidden calories. Fresh, raw ingredients are the key. Easy on the fat and meat, heavy on the vegetables.

RISOTTO

I love risotto and always make one the evening after having a roast chicken to make use of the delicious fresh chicken stock and remaining pieces of meat. It is one of Olly's favorite suppers.

For the base, fry a chopped onion in a smidgen of butter. Cook until soft and translucent. Add Arborio rice and stir for a few seconds, ensuring you coat all the rice in the onion and butter. If you want, you can add a splash of wine at this point, but it's by no means obligatory. Then add boiling chicken stock, ladleful by ladleful, until the rice is cooked but still retains a bit of firmness. Reduce the heat and add some finely grated Parmesan. If you have good chicken stock, this is a delicious meal without any extras.

If you do want to add a bit of razzle-dazzle to it, try adding diced, cooked veggies such as leeks or asparagus. Or you can stir in raw spinach or arugula or meat, if you have any lying around.

Risotto isn't the fastest meal to prepare, but you can cheat and add half the stock immediately over low heat, keep an eye on it, and stir it occasionally rather than constantly as you are supposed to.

FRUIT SALAD

Make up a big bowl of fresh fruit salad at the beginning of the week. Fruit is much more inviting when it's all chopped up and colorful and ready to eat in a big bowl staring out at you every time you open the fridge. Add a splash of fresh orange or apple juice to the mix, and then you can dig into a bowl whenever hunger strikes and only something sweet will do. Add some freshly grated ginger for added zing. Or eat with a dollop of Greek yogurt, but *not* the whole carton.

JUICE

If you're seriously committed to increasing your intake of fruit, I thoroughly recommend getting a juicer.

Try one of the following recipes (being sure to peel and core all necessary ingredients):

- 2 carrots, 1 apple, 1 orange, and a thumb-size piece of ginger

- 2 carrots, 1 apple, 1 kiwi, and a handful of parsley
- 2 apples, half a beet, half a cucumber, and a handful of fresh spinach
- 1 tomato, 2 carrots, 1 celery stick, basil, and the juice of half a lemon

All are totally delicious and put you well on your way to your five a day. Add vodka on a Friday night for a tasty and nutritious cocktail.

THE grit Doctor SAYS

IT'S ALL ABOUT having the right foods ready and accessible—and *not* having access to the wrong ones. It is very difficult even for the Grit Doctor to resist the pull of a box of Girl Scout cookies that's staring out from the cupboard. That wouldn't be an issue if there was only a box of Wasa crispbreads on offer. If you are trying to lose weight, don't have both in the cupboard. Don't punish yourself with choice.

SMOOTHIES

I perfected the art of the smoothie while in France. I had the luxury of a Vitamix there, but a handheld blender is also ideal for the task. I bought stacks of frozen raspberries, strawberries, and other summer berries, which had the double advantages of being cheap and of making the smoothie ice-cold.

The base of a great smoothie is banana. To this, add any number of other ingredients. For dairy-free, fruit-only smoothies add some fruit juice—orange or apple is ideal, but really any juice will do; the purpose is to make the smoothie into a drinkable consistency. Then in go your frozen berries, any number of fresh fruits, or a combination of both. Experiment. I discovered canned pineapples (those in juice, not syrup) are a fantastic ingredient. For a real treat, add a small bowl of vanilla yogurt.

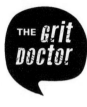

THE grit doctor

WILL SEE YOU NOW

Q: But . . . I'm a busy chef and have to eat at weird times. After work the last thing I want to do is cook again for myself. I know I am eating really badly as I never sit down to a proper meal but snack on pastries and sugary stuff and coffee throughout the day and night to keep me going at work. I have started the running, though, and am really enjoying the "high" I'm getting off it, and I do want to sort this out. HELP!

A: Well done for taking up running. This is the most important step toward shifting your approach to food and you have already taken it. So keep it up, three times a week minimum, five times optimum. Focus on your running "high" as being way better than the old sugar one, and stop using your work as the excuse for maintaining some really bad eating habits. Pastries, sugary stuff, and caffeine are not keeping you going at work. Quite the opposite, in fact. The initial "high" you get from the sugar is followed by a "low," which is what keeps you returning to the cake or substituting with a caffeine hit. Fiber-rich foods like whole grains and fruits will genuinely provide you with the energy you need for your busy job. They release their energy more slowly and make you feel full for longer. Also, be sure to drink a lot more water. These two changes—replacing sugary snacks with fiber-rich ones and drinking more water—will have your energy levels balancing out in no time. Having your big meal early, before your evening shift, will give you that vital energy boost, not to mention a bit of time to yourself. You need to start

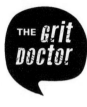

#gritdoctor

GET OFF YOUR ASS AND RUN!

caring about the food you are putting into your mouth at least as much as you care about the food you are putting into the mouths of your customers.

MEAL PLANNING

It's all about knowing what makes up the base of meals. Armed with a good base, you can develop your own recipes to suit your taste preferences and budget and start adapting meals to what you have left in the fridge rather than being tied to a list of obscure ingredients all the time. A good base and the right cooking methods are the foundation upon which to develop your culinary skills.

BASE	HEALTHY ADDITIONS	NAUGHTY TREATS (Save these for special occasions *only**)
Pasta sauce Onions, garlic, fresh tomatoes (or canned if that's what you've got)	Vegetables—as many as you want Fresh herbs Cooked meats, salmon, or tinned tuna A fine shaving of Parmesan	A big handful of grated Cheddar sprinkled over the top
Soup Onions, celery, vegetables of your choice, chicken or vegetable stock	Fresh herbs An artistic swirl of sour cream or a dollop of crème fraîche	Lovely croutons
Stir-fry Onions, garlic, chile peppers, ginger, noodles or rice	Vegetables—as many as you want Prawns, lean chicken, beef, or pork	It's hard to sex up a stir-fry, but you could always add some peanuts or cashews, which are full of fat.

BASE	HEALTHY ADDITIONS	NAUGHTY TREATS (Save these for special occasions *only**)
Risotto Onions, garlic, Arborio rice, chicken or vegetable stock	Mushrooms, butternut squash, or any vegetables you fancy A modest handful of Parmesan	A slightly larger handful of Parmesan, some cream, and a generous glug of white wine during cooking . . . and then a glass for you
Fruit Salad Apples, oranges, bananas, fruit juice	Mango, grapes, kiwi, melon . . . whatever the exotic fruit section of the supermarket has on offer! A small dollop of Greek yogurt	Replace the small dollop of Greek yogurt with a small(ish) dollop of whipped cream
Juice Fruit!	More fruit! Or go crazy and try a vegetable or fresh herbs	Vodka, ice . . . *ahhh*
Smoothies Bananas, fresh apple, orange, or other fruit juice of your choice	Frozen berries, Fresh strawberries, apples, or any other fruit that appeals to you	A bowl of vanilla yogurt—or why not turn your smoothie into a milkshake with some lovely vanilla ice cream?

*Don't become the sort of dull person who invites friends over for dinner and then serves them diet food. If you're on a roll and want to stick to your healthy-eating regime, now is the time to crack open the "luxury" ingredients and add those to your basic recipes. Otherwise, save these for really special occasions only, until you have reached your target weight.

A LITTLE SOMETHING EXTRA FOR THE SEASONED MASOCHIST

Allow yourself to feel real hunger pangs. These may be entirely alien sensations to you. The general advice with any sort of dieting is, of course, the complete opposite: Don't allow yourself to get hungry, and keep your sugar levels up. And no doubt there is a sound basis for this—if you allow yourself to feel really hungry, you are more likely to cave in and binge on sugary junk. However, as a disciplined runner, you are no longer so weak-willed. You are stronger and more determined than the rest. Let yourself feel real hunger pangs, and learn to appreciate them. Recognize when you are *really* hungry, as opposed to just bored, tired, or sad.

Let the feeling last for as long as you feel comfortable, and then eat healthily. Don't give yourself any other option. Don't have fatty foods at home. Don't have sugary treats stocked up in cupboards. Remember, your treat is losing weight through running. Whenever you are tempted to snack or binge on forbidden foods, first look in the mirror, summon your inner bitch, and repeat your mantra. And before you eat anything, drink a glass or two of water. You may find that you are not, in fact, hungry at all.

THE grit doctor SAYS

HUNGER IS OFTEN thirst (FOR WATER) in disguise.

BUT THE grit doctor ALSO SAYS

THERE IS ANOTHER kind of thirst that water cannot quench. Alcohol is fine in moderation. The aim is to work hard, play hard, and look good at all times. The odd Friday night indulgence is to be recommended. The Grit Doctor does not want you to live like a saint. The idea is to get running so that you can enjoy the rest of your life more fully—food, fun, and Friday nights included.

RUNNING ON EMPTY

Running on an empty stomach first thing in the morning is a truly phenomenal experience, especially if you can time it so you run through the sunrise. Keep your clothes and shoes and everything you'll need ready by your bed the night before so you can literally roll out of bed and get into them while still half-asleep. The only other thing you need to do is drink some water, and you are ready to go. **No dawdling.**

If you are anything like me, you will not feel remotely hungry before or during this run. You will instead feel as light as a feather and be able to run so much more easily than at any other time during the day or evening. Nothing sets you up for the day ahead in quite the same way. It will leave you feeling euphoric, unbelievably relaxed, and content, but also incredibly effective and razor-sharp.

A *Grit Doctor* TIP

RUNNING ON EMPTY isn't for everyone, but try it and see before making up your mind.

Running will fundamentally change your relationship with food. You can run on empty and not feel hungry for up to an hour afterward. But when you do feel hungry, you will be ravenous. Soon after a run is the best time to eat, especially if you are trying to lose weight. Your metabolism is at its peak after a run, blood pumping hard through your body, everything working smoothly and efficiently, so you burn off what you eat quickly and easily, much more so than if you had eaten before the run and tried to use it to burn off the calories. Eating before your run will also make it

#gritdoctor

GET OFF YOUR ASS AND RUN!

far less enjoyable as you will feel very heavy and sluggish, making the whole experience feel like more of a trial. So try to run first thing in the morning on an empty stomach if at all possible. Don't panic if you can't—it doesn't matter. I used to run after work in the evenings (before supper, so on an empty stomach) and that worked well for me, too. The morning run is the absolute ideal, with the beach run at sunrise being the mother lode. Do it the next time you're on vacation, and write me a thank-you note.

THE *grit Doctor* SAYS

IF YOU ARE overweight, you are almost certainly eating to fill a hole that is not always about hunger. No amount of food is going to fill it. A run will.

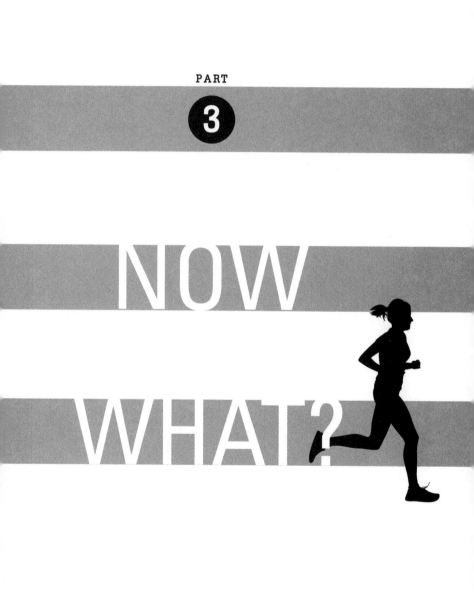

PART

3

NOW
WHAT?

Making It Stick and What to Do When It Won't

Running makes you look good. . . .

When I was pregnant and enjoying that much-fabled "glow," my skin looked remarkably similar to how it used to after a run. It makes perfect sense. When you're pregnant, your blood supply increases and blood is much more visible close to the surface of your skin, contributing to that healthy glow. After a run you glow, too, because your blood is pumping a lot faster around your body and the capillaries close to the surface of your skin have become dilated. And to glow is to be at your most beautiful. Run your way into a glowing complexion, plumped-out skin, and rose-tinted cheeks. This is probably the most effective beauty tip you'll ever be given. No amount of makeup, facials, or even surgery can match the look of your face after a run—the blood so close to the surface of your skin makes it look naturally youthful, and your eyes will sparkle and shine.

S o now you need to turn everything you've learned into a habit. But how? By doing it over and over again. Yes, it is hard. Expect it to be hard. Start digging hard. When bad habits are long ingrained—like eating junk food and remaining glued to the couch—they can be very difficult to shift, BUT SHIFT THEY WILL if we shock ourselves out of them and keep repeating the same healthy routine day in, day out. Beat yourself up when you mess up—be really hard on yourself. The idea is that once your new running and eating regimens become habit—and they will after months of repetition—they won't go away. They will become part of who you are and how you operate. And you will no longer have to think about them or motivate yourself to do them. They will just happen quite naturally as part of your daily routine. I'm talking about running, drinking more water, and taking responsibility for what you put into your body.

Repeating the identical, tried-and-true run day in, day out is precisely the sort of boring habit you need to cultivate in order to guard against motivation meltdown. The more routine the run is, the more effortless it is, until eventually it becomes another part of your day that you no longer have to think about. You will just do it—like bathing and eating—and you won't be derailed by outside forces. The simpler you make it, the easier it will be to cultivate and coax your run into becoming a habit. It becomes more like sleeping and less like going on a date—fraught with decisions and choices about what to wear, where to go, and what to talk about. The fewer choices available, the greater your chance is of simply doing the right thing without thinking about it or trying to worm your way out of it. Yes, it's robotic—that is precisely the idea—but you won't be complaining when you have the body you always dreamed of and can still eat like a king.

MOTIVATION MELTDOWN

It happens. You let your guard down and your motivation suddenly leaves you completely. This is the only real hurdle you will come across in your quest for success—you will wake up knowing that you have to go for a run today, and you won't want to go. You will keep putting it off—"I'll go after lunch," "I'll go this afternoon," "I'll go when I've watched X." The irony is that you won't be able to enjoy X or be productive with the rest of your day until you go on your run. The guilt will grind you down, distracting you from being effective elsewhere.

This guilt is a very important tool to help get you outside. If you miss the occasional run, the guilt gets to you and will probably get you back into your sneakers later the same day or, at the worst, the following day. But when the odd day turns into a couple of months, then you are in real trouble. The guilt will fade, and you are in danger of forgetting everything you have learned. Your running memory is very short where motivation is concerned. The inner bitch that pesters you when you are running regularly is silenced through lack of use. And when that happens, you have lost a valuable motivational aid. That voice is your own personal trainer. Keep your inner bitch talking and that voice will get you into your sneakers and back outside.

This is why it pays to have a set routine for when you go running each day: With a strict routine you can't start playing these pointless mind games with yourself. Your run shouldn't be one of any

MAKING IT STICK AND WHAT TO DO WHEN IT WON'T

number of possible options on any given day but rather an ingrained part of your daily routine. When motivation meltdown strikes, be hard on yourself. With a sense of humor, repeat the "YOU FAT BITCH" routine or your own personal mantra in the mirror, and you should be back outside smiling in no time at all.

The beauty of running is that even if you fall off the wagon—and no matter how long you stay off it—you will still be only two minutes away from having it back in your life again. It doesn't require any retraining or any new extra commitment, but depending on how long you were established in your running routine beforehand, you may require a gentle reintroduction. If you hadn't even completed the Six-Step Program, for example, and fell off the wagon for two weeks, then definitely go back a week or two. Know your limits and be realistic: If you only did a few weeks of the program and then took a year off, you've got to start from scratch. All you need to get started up again are your running shoes and the courage to take those first steps outside.

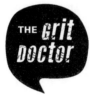

THE grit Doctor WILL SEE YOU NOW

Q: This is my second time trying the Six-Step Program, but running is so boring!

A: Yes, it is boring. Trying to make it a fascinating and fun pursuit will ensure your failure. Embracing the fact that it is boring is one of the keys to your success. Despite this, you may often be pleasantly surprised during the course of a run that the feeling of boredom is replaced by a sense of deep peace and well-being, and you will ALWAYS be glad that you went. ALWAYS.

BE GOAL-CENTRIC

Transform motivation meltdown into motivation zeal by paying to enter a race and pledging to raise a sum of money for charity, ideally one that is of great personal significance. And tell everyone. That way you won't be able to wriggle out of training. Setting yourself goals and putting yourself out there—whether by racing to achieve your personal best, raising money, or beating a friend—are guaranteed to keep you motivated. Check out the Internet and join a club if that's your thing (see Appendix 2, page 197)—or run against work colleagues and beat them. It's all about setting targets—and winning.

THE *grit doctor* SAYS

ANYONE WHO THINKS of running as "fun" does not know the meaning of the word. It is not meant to be fun. If you try to make it fun, you will fail. Fun is what you have after you have been running, and it is what you are because you run.

Ruth . . .

I RECENTLY LOOKED back at something I wrote when I was pregnant and pounding out the first draft of this book. . . .

I was consumed with jealousy watching Olly go about his business this morning having kicked off his day with a run. I want to feel what he is feeling. I want a piece of that endorphin rush. I have to settle for a fast walk each day and I can tell you it is not the same. But my body is being put to a different use for these coming months, and I am determined to enjoy it. But it got me thinking: How will I be able to fit in a run when the twins arrive? This will no doubt be a logistical nightmare, but I simply must find a way. Because I know that the hour I spend pounding Hampstead Heath will be the best hour I can invest in motherhood. It will give me those endorphins I'm desperate for, it will make the more dreary tasks of mothering more tolerable, and it will help me to snatch my sleep wherever I can get it. It will make the whole job that little bit easier to manage and give me energy and patience. And perhaps most importantly, it will help me to enjoy the babies and keep smiling. That's my theory anyway.

—✺—

Ha! Well, now that the twins are nine months old I can be honest about the fact that motivation meltdown struck me in a *big way* after they were born. I'd stopped running for short periods before—a few weeks, a few months even—but nothing like this. This was what I call TOTAL GLOBAL MELTDOWN. My body felt shattered by childbirth. Instead of feeling energized and empowered by the process, I lost all faith in my body. I was afraid of it all the time, afraid it would fail me. My bones seemed somehow to have moved into different positions, and nothing seemed to work properly. There was no way I could run again. I decided instantly that my previous life was over and that I would never have the time or energy to run again. It took every ounce of physical strength I had just to stumble from one day to the next trying to manage with twins. I honestly thought I might die of tiredness. Running was out of the question.

But I kept getting these gently nudging e-mails from my agent about the book, which I had sent her just before the arrival of the twins. The twins were very small and very needy, but I managed to get through the early stages of preparing the book to go out to publishers. I wasn't running, but I was still thinking about running. I couldn't escape it. I tried to go on a run at Christmastime, but it was a disaster and served to confirm all my worst suspicions about my weak and ailing body. It was also bitterly cold, and I was a lot less fit than I thought, probably through a combination of carrying around more weight than I was used to and not having been running in over a year. I became breathless very quickly and had to walk most of my circuit, which was very demoralizing. (Silly, on reflection, to run so soon and in such harsh conditions, too gritty altogether . . . even for the Grit Doctor.) And then, in the new year, my agent told me we had a publishing deal on the table. I was stunned and flabbergasted and felt like a fraud. I hadn't run in eighteen months. I told myself it didn't matter because I had already written the book . . . back when I was a different woman. But the deal came with a request for another twenty thousand words. I found that I had nothing to say. Nothing funny or inspiring or real. I couldn't motivate myself to write at all, let alone write anything good, unless I started running again. And I just couldn't get myself back into it.

It struck me that this place—the place of TOTAL GLOBAL MELTDOWN—is actually the place where lots of people are in the very beginning. A place of no exercise and general apathy. I realized for the first time how very difficult it is to get started. Because after an eighteen-month gap, which included childbirth, my body had retained no running memory, no physical or emotional attachment to the exercise. I even stopped believing that it could be as good as all the things I had written about it. I had gotten used to a new way of being—one of resignation. That it was OK (and of course it *is* OK) to collapse on the sofa with a glass of wine after the twins were down for the night and ask Olly to order some takeout. That eating all that junk didn't really matter. I had stopped caring about my body, though it wasn't getting fat because the twins were burning up everything I had and then some, day after day, week after week, month after month. The bigger they got, the heavier they got, and the more calories I burned, so the more cake and junk I could eat. But I looked awful, and I had no energy at all. I would collapse into bed at nine PM each night and sleep fitfully until one of the babies woke me. But I was so used to this new way of being that I thought, I'm a mom now and this is how it is going to be. No time for anything except the babies, and definitely no time to care about my body.

Two significant things happened, which I guess you could call catalysts. . . .

Catalyst 1: Illness

The twins caught a stomach bug. I caught it from them and was completely knocked down by it. Crawling around the house, cleaning up vomit and diarrhea while unable to keep anything down myself, I was as weak as a kitten. All I could do was cry. No sooner had I recovered from the bug than I came down with an awful cough that required antibiotics and took more than a month to kick. Olly got the cough, too, and needed two courses of antibiotics, inhalers, scans, and all sorts of treatments to get right. I remembered that I never ever used to get ill when I was running. Somehow, running boosts your immune system and seems to guard against catching infections, colds, and the like. Olly and I agreed that looking after the twins was impossible unless we were operating at 100 percent. We both knew that we needed to start running again so that, in turn, we would start looking after our bodies better and caring more about what we were putting into them. Plus, deadlines were fast approaching for submitting the extra text for the book and my word count was a sad few hundred. It was fear, really, for my health, of letting people down, of not getting the job done that got me to stumble outside one spring evening after putting the twins down to bed, Olly just home from work. There was a part of me that was desperate to reclaim something of my former self, some of my old spark, to impress my husband, who had been living with a shadow of the woman he had only recently fallen in love with. I walked to Highgate Wood (about ten minutes, the perfect warm-up), went through the gates, and started up the gentlest of trots. . . .

Catalyst 2: Injury

So Catalyst 1 was enough to get me into my sneakers and out of the front door. I had a slight twinge in my right knee, but fifteen minutes into the run it had disappeared. I ran slowly and deliberately and can honestly say that at no point did I enjoy the run. It was brutal using those muscles again after so long, and it took a gargantuan effort not to stop every five minutes. At no time did I enter any "zone" other than the "Go home NOW and STOP" zone. I was just praying I would complete what I had set out to do—a one-hour run around Highgate Wood. I did. My legs were like lead, and I thought with a start how out of touch with my body I had become. But I felt pretty proud of myself for having completed what I set out to do that day. Getting out of the door once the twins were down, avoiding the fridge and the glass of vino, but using the thought of later treating myself with both to spur me on.

But no sooner had I set foot inside the house again than the magic started. I floated into the kitchen and straight over to the sink. I just wanted water. Gallons of it straight from the tap. It tasted like nectar. I immediately sat down at my computer and started writing. The words came easily and fluently, and before I looked up I had written a thousand words. This is it. It's working. This is the magic that has been missing from my life. I felt energized. I felt happy. I felt exhausted. I fell into bed that night and slept like a log for the first time since the last time I went running. I didn't wake to the tiny noises of the babies, not until the morning— seven thirty AM, in fact, after about ten hours of sleep. It was the longest sleep I'd had since I was about four months pregnant.

I turned to get out of bed, and that's when it happened. My right knee was in agony. I looked at it, a swollen mass of flesh all tender and sore. Come on. I was planning to go running again that evening, write another thousand words, etc.—you get the picture. I had been knocked down at the first hurdle. Lifting the babies and carrying them upstairs is very difficult with the Elephant Man living inside your knee, let me tell you. And I felt so depressed about it. And anxious. Would I be able to write without running? Well, I simply had to. And strangely, I was even more inspired by the fact that I *couldn't* run. It had the same effect as the pregnancy—not being *allowed* to run, rather than *choosing* not to. Somehow, I turned the negative into a positive.

PHONE A FRIEND

Now, I know that earlier I said that "a problem shared is a problem doubled." Well, when you're a brand-new runner, starting out on Step 1 of the Grit Doctor's program, that's certainly true. But if you are a tired and jaded former runner suffering from severe motivation meltdown, it can be really useful to call on the support of your partner or a friend. Get them to be your backup Grit Doctor. It should be someone whose respect you have earned and who you would be mortified to let down. Tell this person that you intend to run and, if necessary, get them to force you out of the door. Brief them beforehand that you have no motivation, that you know you will try everything in the book to get out of it, and that it is their job to ensure that you get outside in your sneakers and do not return for at least an hour. When I was trying to get back into running I used the excuse that I couldn't find my sneakers! Olly found them and put my feet into them and practically laced them up. If, after all that, I had failed to complete my run, the shame would have been too much to bear.

ALWAYS LIE TO YOURSELF

Lying can be a very useful motivating tool when cunningly deployed. I have been getting myself to go on runs lately by telling myself that I will go for a fast walk and run for just 10 minutes and then come home. This gets me out of the door when I simply cannot face going for a run or feel like I don't have the time and my motivation is low. Lying is a great way to get you into your sneakers and outside—which is always the toughest part—forcing you to take those first steps and get through that first awful 10 minutes of *every* run. Because by the time you have done what you set out to do, you will almost certainly want to go farther. If motivation is still low after 10 minutes, tell yourself another lie—just another 5 minutes and then home—and keep increasing the run by small increments if you are still struggling. Before you know it, you have been running for an hour.

Ruth . . .

AFTER I'D SIGNED my book deal, I went into my new publisher's offices to introduce them to the Grit Doctor and give a little talk about the book. I was terrified at the prospect of speaking to a roomful of strangers, which made me feel particularly pathetic given that I am supposed to be a trial attorney used to speaking in court. But presenting to a roomful of strangers (interactive strangers!) is a very different animal from giving a speech to a stone-faced jury (who can't answer back). I spoke to Olly about it the night before and asked his advice about how to get over the nerves. Other than the obvious "go for a run" advice, he suggested owning up to how nervous I was.

I did just that and ended up talking about how running is a great metaphor for life and its challenges. I told them that I was going to approach the talk as I would a run: by doing it even though every part of my body and mind was telling me not to, by expecting the first ten minutes to be hellish and awful and then hoping to warm up a bit thereafter. I was also expecting there to be the odd twinge (and possibly some real pain) during the talk, but I hoped that at the end of it, I would feel really pleased with myself. That's what I said, and it is exactly what happened. It turned out that many of the women in the room were interested in running, and we had a really great, inspiring chat. One of the best areas of discussion was about getting yourself going. How do you turn on that switch to get yourself motivated? Isn't that the million-dollar question, I thought aloud.

I pondered this question for some time after leaving the office. How to flick the switch? And I came to the very gritty conclusion that there simply is *no switch*. Hoping for a switch to be turned on, the lights suddenly to go up and—abracadabra!—there you are, all bright-eyed, bushy-tailed, and raring to go is just like hoping for a pill to make you thin or a knight in shining armor to make you happy. There is nothing you can take or "turn on" to make you take those first steps outside. There is only you and your inner bitch. You have to harness something within yourself and *make* yourself go. YOU CAN DO IT.

How to Recover Your Running Mojo Post-Baby/Injury/Illness— And Why Running Is Better Than Therapy

Running tunes your internal bullshit meter. . . .
Once you have got off your ass and completed the circuit that you thought you never could when you started out, you will realize that you can apply the same gritty approach to everything else in your life that you resist. Think how long you fought against exercise and healthy eating. Consider the other stuff you may be resisting: changing jobs, dealing with relationship issues, cleaning your house, for example. Through the practice of running, you will become less tolerant of the nonsense that stops you from facing up to difficult stuff, and deal with it instead. It's probably due to a combination of the physiological "happy" effect and a shift in attitude. But whatever the reason, running makes you tolerate less of your own bullshit, let alone other people's. And that is a very good thing.

C oming back to running after a long absence can be just as daunting as starting out for the first time. I experienced this firsthand post-pregnancy, but there are all sorts of other physical problems, illnesses, and injuries from which coming back to running can require Herculean amounts of grit. Ultimately, the solution always involves accessing your inner bitch and harnessing her voice to divert you away from the couch and get you outside in your sneakers again instead. Once you are there—outdoors in your sneakers—90 percent of the job is done. Sharing stories about getting back into the running groove is often the best medicine to give other "almost ex-" runners just the nudge they need to push themselves back out there.

Ruth . . .

I THOUGHT I should write a bit about my own experiences of the effect of pregnancy and childbirth on my runner's body and how I am dealing with it. Because I am still dealing with it. The advice and tips in this section, however, are equally applicable to all runners who have been derailed by other physical setbacks, serious injury, or illness.

POST-CHILDBIRTH RUNNING

The number one rule is this: Do not go for a run too soon after childbirth—especially if you have had a C-section. I realize this should be obvious, but in my opinion the six-week no-exercise rule should be extended considerably when it comes to running. And this advice obviously applies to *any* serious operation. Your body has been through the equivalent of a car crash and needs time to repair itself. The body needs rest to heal; the bones that shifted and the muscles that softened and relaxed in preparation for childbirth need time to adjust and strengthen again. And this applies to other injuries as well. There is nothing more counterproductive in running terms than rushing back into it after an injury or illness, no matter how big or small. A sprained ankle run on too soon can become a broken one, requiring months to heal. Similarly, a body recovering from major surgery needs time to recuperate, and a run too soon will not "speed up" the recovery process.

THE *grit Doctor* SAYS

DON'T TRY TO run before you can walk.

I was honestly afraid that everything might fall out—I felt very tender and protective of my womb area and nether regions. The hormone relaxin softens all the muscles of the pelvic floor to allow your body to endure childbirth, and your womb obviously has to deflate thereafter, so that area feels very strange—entirely foreign, in fact—for some time after delivery. Don't underestimate how fragile and tender you may feel for a while down there. Jumping up and down too soon (like I did) may put you off it for good (as it nearly did to me).

Before you start any running at all, make sure you have been doing a lot of walking—ideally pushing your stroller, which is a great workout in itself and will slowly build up your fitness for that first run. And it's not just fitness that you need to build up. It's confidence. That was a real problem for me after having the twins. After a very traumatic birth, I was left feeling that my body was not up to any exercise and certainly not up to running.

First-timers

For the first-time runner who is also a first-time mom, you can just follow the program in Chapter 3 (page 47), taking along your stroller to establish the circuit if you wish. But *don't run with the stroller* until you are an established runner. Once you have an established running routine and feel the need to challenge yourself, feel free to join the pushy parent brigade and kill two birds with one stone: Get your baby outside for some fresh air and give yourself a fantastic workout. Be sure to use an appropriate stroller—i.e., one that is designed to allow you to run and push. NOT YOU, MOTHERS OF MULTIPLES. It is not safe to run with your double stroller, nor remotely sane, and you absolutely need to get away from those babies for your run. The Grit Doctor's orders.

It is perfectly safe to run while breastfeeding (obviously not actually *during* a breastfeed), but you will need to take extra care with nutrition and hydration. Simply put, eat more and drink more water. The right bra is crucial and, of course, nursing pads can help deal with leakage.

I would actually suggest waiting until your baby is sleeping through the night before you start running. Maybe I am less gritty than I thought, but I tried to run three months in and was so exhausted afterward that I found the night shift almost impossible. Perhaps if I'd carried on it would have been different, but that one run too soon put me off trying again for another three months.

Old-timers

If you ran before your pregnancy, you should expect to feel different after it, so don't expect to be able to go at it full-force like you did before you had babies. Not straightaway, that is. However, you are the best judge of your limits. Go for a short, slow run, and take your temperature—metaphorically speaking—once you have been given the all-clear by your doctor. If you are a Paula Radcliffe type, clearly you will be able to run a marathon and win it very soon thereafter. Having a baby is no reason or excuse to think you are not up to it anymore. You absolutely are, and you may well enjoy the happiest, sexiest time of your life post-babies. Not only that, you may end up with an even better body. And do take full advantage of that feeling that you can conquer the world because you survived giving birth to fuel your running addiction and lust for life. You can do anything and you will transform that desire into action through a committed running practice. Just be prepared for your body to feel a bit different now.

THE *grit doctor* SAYS

YOU MAY BE lacking in iron and calcium post-childbirth, so take a supplement if necessary. It will become another thing that you are doing for yourself in taking care of your body, which is a very positive thing indeed.

Postpartum Depression

For the love of God, look after yourself and do what your real doctor tells you—not the Grit Doctor. I was really down for a long time after the twins were born. The sleep deprivation was probably the main cause, but I now realize that the lack of exercise was also a major factor. The twins were born in late September, so those early months were pretty grim, night feeds in the dark and early morning starts in the dark—hideous. My motivation and confidence were at an all-time low. Postpartum depression, however, is a very serious condition that requires help, treatment, and medication. Notwithstanding this, if you have been diagnosed with postpartum depression (no self-diagnosis, please), do ask your doctor if you can start the Six-Step Program. My feeling is that it would be wholeheartedly endorsed as very good therapy indeed.

MY TOP TIPS FOR GETTING OUT THERE AGAIN AFTER A LONG-TERM ABSENCE

- I get into my running clothes and sneakers during the afternoon when I've put the twins down for a nap so I am mentally prepared to head out of the door once they are asleep.
- I text Olly during the afternoon and tell him I want to go for a run the minute he gets home and to make me go if I try to wriggle out of it. He is my backup Grit Doctor.
- I plan something totally delicious and massive for dinner as a reward and get Olly involved in preparing it while I am out running and fantasize about it during the run. Or I heat something up the moment I return from my run that I already prepared the night before so it is ready to eat when I get out of the shower.
- I lie to myself. As mentioned earlier, the hour's run in 10-minute increments is a cunning trick to get me out of the door in the first place and then all the way around my route.

- Throughout the day I want to go running and during the run itself I repeat this mantra, stolen from a great friend who supplied a case study for the book: *Every time you run, you win. Even a bad run is a win. Small win after small win. Day after day. WHEN YOU RUN, RUTH, YOU WIN.* It gives me shivers up and down my spine and propels me forward. Use it or find one of your own: a pithy line that gets you going and fires you up. "RUN, FAT BITCH, RUN" always works for me.

And think of all the benefits you'll get from just *leaving the house* and stretching your body and mind.

- Freedom from all your responsibilities. It is temporary (unless you keep on running, but I'm not for one moment suggesting that, however tempting it might sometimes seem!), but it feels amazing that for an hour you can be completely on your own again.
- Rediscovery of yourself as a person beyond your work and family roles.
- Resculpting all of the muscles and body tone lost since childbirth.
- Creative thinking.
- A sense of incredible peace.
- Exploring the beauty of nature and your local community without the stroller. Taking in all the nooks and crannies that it prevents you from getting to.
- Unbeatable fat-burning exercise and cardio workout.
- A phenomenal night's sleep during which you won't wake to every tiny noise that the baby makes.
- Renewed confidence and motivation as a mother.

- Increased love and patience for your baby and partner.
- Energy to do all of your chores and enjoy looking after the baby.
- Enhanced sexual drive along with the increased energy and appetite for life!
- Determination to go running again and continue improving in all areas.

That hour is YOU time. You won't be able to fill this hour with mothering or wife-ing (which you *will do* if you stay indoors). It's all about *you* for an hour—for once! For your thoughts. For your body. For your mind. And it works. It really works. You'll come back refreshed and happy. Feeling more loving toward your partner, and seeing your baby again for the miracle he or she is. And you will start to take care of yourself again after the experience of having your body and mental well-being taken over by the baby's needs. It is truly awesome. But the Grit Doctor accepts that it requires an awesome amount of effort, too.

Convert whatever inspiration you can find into motivation fuel for your running tank. Thinking about others overcoming greater obstacles than those you face can be just the ticket to get you running again after a long absence.

To: The Grit Doctor
From: Toby
Re: My Running Comeback

I was a keen runner for many years until I was diagnosed with cancer two years ago and had to have a kidney removed. The effect of the cancer treatment was incredibly debilitating and the aftermath of a general anesthetic knocked me sideways. I became bloated and depressed and spent a lot of time sitting on the couch and feeling sorry for myself.

I did think about running, but for the life of me couldn't remember how on earth I ever motivated myself to get out there and actually do it. My wife kept telling me to give it a go, that I would feel so much better. I knew she had my best interest in mind but still I couldn't get myself going again. It was as though the illness had completely robbed me of any motivation to exercise or look after myself. Then one day, my wife gave me an article to read about someone coming back to professional sports after a terrible accident that had left them all but paralyzed. It was such an inspiring story about overcoming all the odds and suddenly I felt terribly ashamed of myself. Here I was with my health and strength back and instead of celebrating it I was wallowing in a sea of misery all of my own creation.

It was the sense of shame that got me to put on my sneakers again for the first time. It was hard. I won't pretend it was easy; my fitness level was considerably less than before, but I knew that it would come back if I just kept at it, step by step, mile by mile, week by week. I am pleased to say that a year later I am back to old running form and looking forward to my fifth marathon in October. ■

RUN FOR YOUR LIFE

Running can help you cope with all sorts of struggles. A great friend of mine, who I knew had taken up running in the last few years, wrote a very moving account of how running helped her during a tremendously difficult time.

The secret I kept hidden was that I started running as an escape. The escape was psychological as well as physical: not from the insistent demands of a baby and toddler as everyone assumed, not particularly as an escape from the effects on my body of two pregnancies and too much food, but as an escape from the crushing weight of domestic abuse.

Always conscious of my size (often described as "robust"), I saw my figure as a battleground and I was rarely the victor. A moment of enlightenment came when, with the children in the bike trailer, I almost failed to go half a mile, halted by the mildest incline which would not even merit the word *hill*. At the same time, my marriage was coming back into focus after the distractions of babies, a move, and new job. In reality, the patterns of abuse had always been there, subtly in the background. The immediate pressures of working parenthood were just increasing the difficulties, and my determination to be the best mother I could, and work to the best of my abilities, meant that my husband's sense of displacement was coupled with anger and aggression. Aggression that ranged from passive to most certainly active. I was frequently told I was fat and unattractive and sex became an area of increasingly hostile discontent. So, a part of the plan to "sort out" of the marriage was to remedy the "fat" side of things and I hoped that losing weight, along with a barrage of other strategies, would change my husband's behavior.

So I started running, only because it was the most exercise I could do in the shortest time away from the children and the house. The smallest circuit was one and a half miles and a stitch would inevitably come within the first half mile. Then the stitch would come later, then the circuit was stitch-free. Next came a longer route—three miles with a hill—then six miles became the staple circuit, and so it built up. With longer runs, I escaped more and felt mentally free. But with longer runs, the anger increased and I was faced with the choice of a run plus anger, a longer run plus more anger, or no run, and discontentment and still anger from my husband.

At one point, my husband said it was like I was having an affair. Only the affair was with running. The evidence? He fixed me with a steely stare, felt under the bed, and brandished his evidence. *Runner's World* magazine.

The more I ran, the more anger and abuse I was escaping from. The crunch came when I began a weekly half-marathon circuit. Two hours, I was told, was not acceptable. Nine hours of golf was, apparently, perfectly fine.

I sought counseling but then I was banned from going by my husband. The counselor had picked up on the abuse instantly and advised me to get out of the marriage for the safety of the children. The situation would inevitably spiral down, she said.

Thinking I could change the situation, and with some resentment, I decreased my running and tried another series of marriage-saving strategies. But the desire to run, to escape, remained. As predicted, things spiraled: the anger exploded, the abuse worsened. Running became my only coping mechanism, my natural Prozac, and I came to rely completely on its power of escape and its effects psychologically and physiologically.

My now ex-husband finally left and once the locks were

changed, the feeling of safely seeped back into my life—a feeling too underappreciated in my earlier life that I still revel in. It's a feeling similar to the high of running: that you are free, that you are uninhibited and you could keep running forever. ▪

I recently met up with this friend. She is still going through a fairly messy divorce but is coping brilliantly and is using running to help keep her sane. Whatever difficult circumstances exist, whatever issues you are dealing with, and whatever mental battles you are fighting, running can be hugely helpful to see you through tough times. Not only does it provide the space and time for constructive thinking, but the endorphins generated will also make you feel better about whatever it is that is troubling you, too.

HOW RUNNING CAN CURE HEARTACHE

Nothing cures a broken heart like a good run. I ran my way through the pain after being dumped one Christmas Eve and came out the other side in springtime looking and feeling great. A run will inevitably make you feel less sad and less deranged (because of the happy hormones). Equally, in running you are caring for your body in a way that heartbreak might otherwise prevent you from doing. Instead of starving or binging and wallowing or drinking yourself into an early grave, by running you are cherishing your body and bruised heart. In keeping fit and looking good you will give your self-confidence a much needed boost. My sister's best friend, Polly, recently told me that running has cured her heartbreak—well, almost.

I can't sleep, I don't feel hungry, I can't set my mind to anything for more than a few minutes, my whole body hurts and I feel sick. And then I run. Running is the best antidote to heartbreak I've ever known.

When I run I can focus my mind in the most rational way; I don't overthink and as I focus on putting one foot in front of the other, I can order my feelings about him and the panic subsides. Equally, I can let all thoughts of him fall out of my mind, empty my head, and think of nothing at all except the sound of my breathing and footsteps and snippets of strangers' conversations.

Running is the purest way I have found to deal with the seemingly endless ache. The pain doesn't go away completely but it is far more bearable and I am, at least, starving and physically exhausted rather than numb when I run every day. I feel so lively when I've done my few miles and I look forward to the next day when I can get the rush again—it's the healthiest addiction I've ever had. And I hope that if and when I ever see him again, I will look incredible. ■

And she does—look incredible, that is.

When the Addiction Takes Hold

Running teaches you to enjoy your own company. . . .

This is something that my husband pointed out to me recently, that he has really started to relish that time on his own (time away from the Grit Doctor, perhaps?). Some of you may already be lovers of your own company—I certainly am—in which case there is nothing better than getting to indulge that side of your personality, whenever you feel the urge, by going off for a run. This can be especially handy if you are in a situation with loads of people and need to escape. No one is going to criticize you for going off for a run (they might if you snuck off to a bar without inviting anyone). I'm thinking Christmas at home, surrounded by family and friends when you're frankly sick to death of all of them. Go for a run, and not only will that hour be pure heaven, but it will also give you the strength and patience to deal with the rest of your time at home. Better still, you may actually relax and enjoy it.

SHARE THE LOVE, BUT BEWARE THE *OVER*SHARE

For God's sake, don't talk about running all the time. I know I am, but I am writing a book to help you. You wouldn't, however, catch me talking about this stuff at a dinner party. Food and exercise talk is very low-grade chat. Much more interesting and inspiring to just *be* the amazing person you have become through running: contented, peaceful, energized, and invigorating company. Be sure to try to encourage and motivate others, but not by lecturing. Buy this book for your friend instead and spread the word that way. Wait until someone notices that you look a whole lot better—thinner and happier—and only then, casually mention what you are doing:

> "Thanks. Actually, I've taken up running."
> "Wow, how did you get started?"
> "Well, it was surprisingly easy. I read this amazing book and just got started, really."

And leave it at that. Don't shove it down people's throats. Let them ask for help first. There are three obvious exceptions to the "don't talk about it" rule. Obviously, it's a good idea to spill the beans over a deep and meaningful catch-up with your best friend. The second exception is before, during, and after a race with fellow competitors. The third is if you ever find yourself at a dinner party made up entirely of fanatical runners. Go for it. Unleash the beast. Who knows where it might lead. . . .

If you're an avid runner living with a bona fide couch potato, the temptation to evangelize about the benefits of running can be too much to bear. I definitely *over*shared my running enthusiasm when Olly and I first met and totally put him off. But eventually I figured out that subtle demonstrations of the benefits of running were far more effective that lecturing him, and he is now, as we have seen, transforming into a lean, mean running machine. Quality "sharing," delivered the right way at the right time, is nothing short of an art form—the deployment of which requires great skill and ingenuity. Get it wrong and you lose your audience. Get it right, however, and you can change lives. What follows is what I recommend if you share your life with a long-term exercise-phobe.

- **Do *not*** manically bang on about the benefits of running. It will do nothing to convert the nonbeliever. Olly thought it was very weird, cultlike, and boring to hear any running talk whatsoever and made that clear very early on in our relationship.
- **Do** exploit opportunities to stand next to him/her naked in the mirror (remember, delusions of *thinneur* are doubly true when you are in denial and are overweight). Resist the urge to make comments, but do stand in such a way that accentuates as much as possible the differences between you.
- **Do** continue running and slyly *demonstrate*, rather than advocate, in as many ways as you can the many post-run benefits. For example: improved mood, sleeping like a log, eating like a horse, having an insatiable sexual appetite.
- **Do** take advantage of any opportunity to drink gallons of water in front of him/her while pretending to enjoy it and making appropriate noises of appreciation.

- **Do** lead by example on the food front. Always make healthy food choices in your partner's company and eat to your heart's content. It will no doubt irritate and confuse him/her enormously that you seem to eat as much, if not more, than he/she does, yet remain super-toned. Gently explain that you go running every day, which burns off a lot of fuel, and that's why you can eat so much, and that it's great, isn't it!

- **Do** *not* forget his/her pride. Don't emphasize your infinite superiority in such a way that might be humiliating—this is likely to put him/her off for good (from running *and* from you).

- **Do** encourage him/her *when it's deserved,* and give appropriate honest compliments. And when he/she tells you what a beautiful, toned, slim, fit body you have, do not respond by telling him/her the same thing if it isn't true. Instead say, "You could, too, darling. It's just because I run. It keeps me in such good shape."

- **Do** set the best possible example by sticking to your running routine and demonstrating your self-discipline in other areas of your life. When asked, always acknowledge that running is the reason why. Before long, and with a bit of luck, your other half will be so inspired by you that he/she will join the club. If inspiration fails, then competition may win the day, because no one likes to be outshone by his/her other half. In the end he/she will want a piece of the action.

#gridoctor **GET OFF YOUR ASS AND RUN!**

> THE GRIT DOCTOR is all for pushing yourself further, stepping outside of
> your comfort zone, and becoming the best version of yourself. Some of you
> will get obsessed with running and the Grit Doctor is eager for you to take
> advantage of this zeal.

ADVANCED RUNNING

Remember, all of you who have completed the Six-Step Program
and are able to run for 45 minutes without stopping at least three
times a week are more than ready to enter a 5K race. DO IT. Racing
is amazing and so motivating. There will be numerous local 5Ks you
can enter (see Appendix 2, page 197, or ask at your local running
store). Now is a great time to rope in a friend—maybe someone you
know who is a runner but who doesn't yet know you are? Invite him
or her to enter a 5K race with you. Just stick to what you are doing,
running regularly, and that is all the training you need to do. Unless,
of course, you plan on winning the race, in which case work through
the training program that follows and run like the wind on race day.

INCREASING DISTANCES

Now that you are so much fitter and able to complete your circuit
easily (and, crucially, in less time), you can squeeze in some extra
mileage. You should be able to go from a 3- or 4-mile run to a 4- or
5-mile run quite effortlessly and enjoy the extra high you will get
from your regular run. Don't attempt to progress from a 4-mile to an

8-mile run overnight. Use the same strategies for increasing distance you employed during the Six-Step Program—slow and steady all the way.

Fitting in a long run over the weekend is a great way to increase your fitness and stamina. An 8-miler will really satisfy your running lust and take you to a whole new world of satisfaction.

If you are desperate to escape a dull running route, there is no harm in locating a nearby green area, hopping in your car or jumping on a bus, and treating yourself to a run in more scenic surroundings. This is also a good excuse for extending your distance. Mapping the run in advance will help you create a longer circuit, and hopefully the beauty of your surroundings will distract you from the pain in your calves.

INCREASING SPEED

Another good way to challenge yourself to greater heights is increasing your speed. This can be done in a couple of ways: by increasing your overall speed so you complete your circuit in less time or by using interval training. No need to get overly complicated about it, either.

Speed training is essential for improving times and is also great for burning fat. If you start reading running Web sites and "proper" running books, they'll call it either tempo training, fartlek (don't panic—it's Swedish for speed training), or interval training. In essence, it means intervals of running fast and then jogging slowly to recover. It can get incredibly complicated if you try to monitor this while following specific distances unless you are doing laps of a proper racing track. In which case, great—one fast lap followed by one slow recovery lap, and repeat.

FOOLING AROUND WITH stopwatches is generally better for wasting time than tracking it. Just mix up your speed during your regular runs and don't worry about the exact times.

The easiest way to incorporate some speed training into your running regimen is simply to run your already well-established circuit using your knowledge of your route to extend and improve upon your speed. Tell yourself, "Right, I will sprint to that tree," then run slowly to that bench. Run fast, then run slow, then run fast, then run slowly again. Or run fast while counting to 100 in your head, then slow while counting to 100 as I do. The aim is always that the recovery time shortens as you get fitter. You can use a stopwatch if you have one and are able to use it effectively to motivate yourself and monitor your progress, as opposed to letting it distract you and deter you from making progress.

Ruth . . .

IN FRANCE, HEAVILY pregnant and letting out all my frustrations on my poor husband, I insisted Olly do some speed work to increase his fitness once he was running confidently through his circuit. There was a soccer field in our village, and I took Olly there to do interval training. It was so much fun. For me. Standing in the middle of the field, trying not to fall over, I screamed, "SPRINT. STOP. JOG."

SPRINT. STOP. JOG. I must have looked and sounded like a madwoman about to give birth to a whale . . . possibly in the act of giving birth to a whale. The villagers stopped and stared, and many laughed, but Olly was very good. By this stage he had become very fit indeed, and I was a very proud wife.

Once I'd cracked my original circuit, it gave me the confidence to start seeking out different routes and really explore the countryside around the village. I ran down every road or pathway that I could find, just to see where it would take me. Along the way I'd peer into people's houses, speculate wildly on their jobs and relationships, and generally have a good look around.

I found a great run which took me past a grand-looking château and up through some woods to ruins on the outskirts of town, and another which took me past an abandoned Renault parked in a ditch, a field full of horses, and a converted chapel. Such was my sudden desire to push myself that I even got Ruth to take me to the local soccer field and do interval training with me. In other words, she stood in the middle of the field while I ran around the edge and every so often shouted "SPRINT!" at me. I actually enjoyed it. Although not, I suspect, quite as much as Ruth did. ■

HILL TRAINING

Not for the fainthearted, hill training is a great way to test your stamina and endurance, to give you an unbelievable sense of achievement and possibly a spectacular view from the top. The Grit Doctor's favorite.

RUN OFF THE BEATEN PATH

Go somewhere completely different. Plan a new run beforehand. Take in more cross-country. You don't need to follow anything other than your animal instinct for increased fitness and challenges. Go for it. Exploring all the nooks and crannies in the quest for the perfect running circuit can fill you with the spirit of an intrepid explorer. You also will become more rooted in your local community through running, be that a city or the middle of nowhere. Running can force you out of your routine and enable you to appreciate and connect with your environment.

This can help stave off motivation meltdown, but don't get complacent. It will still hit you. YES. IT. WILL. Sometimes the higher you've climbed, the farther you have to fall. So never take it for granted. Remember the importance of routine in your daily running regimen, but by all means go crazy once in a while, or when you're visiting somewhere new. Otherwise, try to keep to your established route on your regular runs.

To: The Grit Doctor
From: Father Henry Wansbrough
Re: Extreme Running

I used to coach rugby and athletics at the monastery attached to the school where I taught, and after athletics in the summer we would often run over to the lake on the edge of the school grounds as a wind down and have a swim. On other days I got into the habit of going for a run by myself. That is when I do a lot of my thinking, preparing lectures or classes. It is lovely countryside with great views and I find the solitude and tranquility very healing.

There are some woods nearby with a thousand different paths—I can still get lost there after running in them for over fifty years. That adds an element of excitement. When I go to lecture or teach in other monasteries it is very relaxing to get out and away from everything and explore the countryside—after a few days I often find I know it better than the inhabitants themselves, though I only go about five to eight miles. Again there is a certain amount of adventure. In Kenya I was almost attacked by a buffalo. In Zimbabwe I ran up the Zambezi, got hot and dove in for a swim, quite unaware that it was full of crocodiles. In the US I went running in the morning on a broad empty road and then as the traffic built up discovered that it was an interstate highway.

I suppose the most important thing which starts me up again is the need for solitude and simply the enjoyment of the grass, the wild flowers, and the trees. It is said that there are puma in those woods, too. . . . ■

Father Wansbrough, who used to teach my brothers, is eighty years old and still runs most days.

CONCRETE ADVICE

The reason that running on concrete *seems* so much easier is because it is, in fact, much easier. You bounce straight off it almost as soon as your feet touch the ground. To the novice this can be seductive, but for all the wrong reasons. You will be able to go for longer and won't feel so tired so quickly, which is why it is very important not to get fooled by the concrete in the early stages of your running career. Run on the softer surfaces: Grass is the best, trails and dirt tracks a close second. Yes, it feels difficult. Yes, it is hard. Hard is the new black, remember? (Repeat this to yourself as you get stuck in the mud.) One day you may be able to run barefoot on sand. As I have already mentioned, running on an empty beach at sunrise or sunset is an incredible experience. But it is not something for the novice runner because the give from the sand makes for a profoundly intensive workout for your legs. The ache in those calves and butt is like nothing you have ever known.

THE grit Doctor WILL SEE YOU NOW

Q: I live in the city and want to run, but I think I have weak knees, so I'm afraid to run on concrete. I do have a gym membership, though, which I rarely use. Is it OK to run on the treadmill?

A: First, please have your knees checked out by a doctor to get a proper diagnosis. There is a wide range of knee-strengthening exercises you can do that might ameliorate the problem. Some knee problems can be all but cured by wearing a proper pair of orthotics or sneakers.

The "dreadmill" is, unsurprisingly, not a piece of equipment the Grit Doctor favors. Running on a conveyor belt like a hamster on a wheel under artificial lighting while your eyes are glued to MTV for distraction goes completely against the Grit Doctor grain. However, the treadmill is great in an emergency.

Emergency situations include:

- Weather conditions so extreme as to make outdoor running impossible and incredibly dangerous (hailstones the size of golf balls, hurricane winds, etc.). Slipping on black ice and breaking an ankle will just put you back on your ass where you started.

- Recovering from a knee or ankle injury—because treadmills are easier on the joints.

Look, if the choice is between staying on the couch and running on the treadmill, then, of course, it's the treadmill every time. While you are there, and once you have gotten up and running, make use of your gym membership to improve on your all-around body tone and fitness with core-strengthening exercises, cross-training, weights, etc. By the time your membership is due for renewal, you will be stronger and fitter and hopefully those knees will be ready to get outside for an airing. I want you to embrace the great outdoors and take control of your fitness using everything you have already.

When your gym membership comes up for renewal, *cancel it*—and spend the money on high-quality sneakers. Wearing them, take all that you have learned on the treadmill out onto the streets. You will never look back.

A REMINDER FROM THE *Grit Doctor*

THE GRIT DOCTOR wants you to win. The great thing about running is that just by setting out on a run, every time you put one foot in front of the other, you win. And entering a race is a big win. In committing to the race and training program you have already won. After that, it's up to you what constitutes a win. Set a time for yourself. Try to outdo a friend—or the person running just a bit in front of you at the end. See how many people you can overtake. That sort of thing. All are wins. *Every time you put one foot in front of the other you win—that is the beauty of running.*

Ruth . . .

WHEN I TOLD my mother that I was running the London Marathon, she got herself a bit worked up about it, which I thought was weird. She didn't want to come to London to watch me run—she said she was too nervous—and it was only the night before the marathon that I discovered why. She called me up and burst out:

"Darling, promise me one thing?"

"What, Mum?"

"That you won't try and win it."

Unbelievable. My mother had visions of me up in the front trying to overtake Paula Radcliffe. I wish. I was bemused and very flattered. Such is my competitive streak that my mother could not imagine my entering a race and not trying to win it. She then complained bitterly afterward that she hadn't seen me on the TV. Clearly she had been looking in all the wrong places—in other words, a few paces behind Paula.

OPTIONAL EXTRAS FOR ADDED GRIT FACTOR

THE GRIT DOCTOR does not want you to get sidetracked by other exercises in the early stages of your running program (because of the inevitable time-wasting involved), but once you've mastered the running and are trying to push yourself, and if you are tough enough, then doing some sit-ups, push-ups, and pull-ups at the end of your run is fantastic. Yes, just lie down on a patch of grass and get on with it. This will help strengthen and improve core muscle groups, which ultimately will improve your running. You will also look hard as nails.

FOOD AND DRINK

If you're training more, eat more—if you feel like it. You can, because you will be burning it off. Drink more water. And take water on your long run. Remember that, even on race day, sports drinks are unnecessary for training at this level and will only add a huge number of wasted calories to your daily intake—calories that would be better spent on a massive meal and a few celebratory drinks afterward. But straight after the race DRINK MORE WATER.

The Grit Doctor's 10K Training Plan

Running boosts your confidence. . . .

This was a benefit I certainly had not anticipated when I took up running, but it is very real. And it doesn't just come from the better body you get that you will be eager to show off. You will start to feel confident in all other areas of your life—at work and on dates, for example. In fact, confidence is one of the best side effects of running. Good self-esteem and confidence are the bedrocks of happiness and success, after all. (They also enable you to make better friends with your inner bitch.) With confidence, your life opens up and the possibilities are endless. Sounds unbelievably cheesy, I know. But it's true.

Slow Coaches, do not get depressed at the thought that a 10K race will never be possible for you, particularly if you are reading this book straight through and have not yet left the couch. Trust me, once you have the six steps under your belt, you will find yourself coming back to this plan, because before long, 5K is going to be too *easy*. For you Fast Trackers, this may be just the challenge you are ready for right now, and if that is the case, read on.

THE *Grit Doctor* RECOMMENDS

USE YOUR WORKWEEK as a template to train for the 10K, using the weekdays for your serious training, with a very important exception: Do not make Monday the worst day. (Mondageddon is not the way to start any week. Even the Grit Doctor always eases herself into a Monday.) Take Friday as your rest day, Saturday as your long run day, and Sunday for your easy run—that way you still get a bit of a weekend. Don't feel you have to follow this slavishly; remember to use your initiative and adapt schedules to suit yourself. Just be sure to take a rest day, but don't overdo it—the resting, that is. And always keep in tune with that body of yours—listen to it carefully and stick to the grass and trails as much as you can.

A 10K is equivalent to 6.2 miles, and unless you are superhuman, this is farther than you have been running thus far during your 45-minute, thrice-weekly jog. You could run it without training if you just continued to run as you are, but in order to enjoy it and stretch yourself, I recommend stepping up your

#gritdoctor ⬩ GET OFF YOUR ASS AND RUN!

regimen. What follows is a rough guide for what I did when training to run in a 10K a few years back. For some serious motivation, sign up for a race 8 weeks from *right now*, and get started on the plan immediately.

THE *Grit Doctor* SAYS

IT IS NOT a train crash if you miss a session, or swap sessions, or change your rest days—the keys to success at 10K are doing some interval training to improve your stamina and speed and getting a longer run in each week to increase your distances. Try to incorporate some hill running into your longer weekend run if possible as this is a fantastic way to improve your powers of endurance.

WEEK 1

MONDAY

If possible, do some exercise today other than running: cross-training, swimming, or a sexathon are all perfect. If this is impossible because you burned your gym membership (the Grit Doctor applauds you for this) or do not have a willing partner, don't worry. Other types of exercise are in no way crucial to your success at a 10K. Go on a very short run or a long walk and/or have a good rest. Mondays are essentially Fundays to be spent as you wish. The grit begins tomorrow.

TUESDAY

As with all running, interval training requires you to warm up first, so do your usual brisk walk to get your muscles relaxed. And then run those first 10 minutes at your usual pace to get yourself into the run. Then run fast for the first 100 meters and then run the next 100 meters really slowly to recover, then go fast again, and then go slow again. If you do not have access to a running track, do not panic. It does not matter. Just go for your normal run and try to run roughly 100 meters fast (just count up to 100 in your head while running or count 100 of your steps, and that will do nicely) and then go slowly for the next 100 meters to recover. Repeat, running in total two fast and two slow stints (4 x 100 meters). Then run the remainder of your run at your usual pace, making up the full 45 minutes. Well done! This is really hard the first time you do it.

THE *grit doctor* SAYS

FOR THE FIRST-TIMER, interval training makes "hard is the new black" look even blacker. But you are going to learn to LOVE it.

WEDNESDAY

Forty-five minutes of easy running. By that I mean your usual 45-minute run. Start to think of your "easy" run as a welcome break from the slightly more gritty training sessions. It should be second nature to you by now and a "pleasure" in the Grit Doctor sense of the word.

THURSDAY

Interval training again as per Tuesday. If you want to vary your interval session, or simply cannot face a repeat performance of Tuesday's grit-fest, you can swap it for a hill session. This involves incorporating a hill into your 45-minute run and, as you move through the weeks and get closer to race day, running up it faster. If you are turning into a grit-fiend, do feel free to combine the two within the same training session: sprints and hills.

FRIDAY

Rest, relax, and enjoy yourself. I'm sure you already know how to do this just fine.

THE grit Doctor WILL SEE YOU NOW

Q: I am training for a 10K and can get myself out of the door no problem on the weekends, but during the week the only time I have to run is before work. I have been setting my alarm for six AM each day, only to turn it off and go back to sleep. Any tips on how to summon up the extra grit to get myself out of bed at six AM?

A: Once roused from sleep, your inner bitch loves nothing more than a run at sunrise. She is not, however, so keen on hearing the alarm clock. Accept that you are never going to hear your alarm and "feel" like jumping out of bed and going for a run. To to get up at five thirty AM to go running before work, you may find you have to set your mobile phone alarm to a much more gritty, in-your-face sort of wake-up call than the usual gentle one—and leave said alarm out of reach of the bed so you have to get out of bed to turn it off. Getting out of your bed is nine-tenths of the battle. Then pull on your running clothes (which you must leave out and ready the night before) and head straight outside, stopping only at the tap to drink a glass or two of water. I was honestly still half-asleep during this process, which worked well for me, as the run had begun before I could question the insanity of getting up so early. Nothing compares to running through the break of dawn—you will feel so proud of yourself all day, and you will feel unbelievably good when you arrive at work. Plus, breakfast will quite literally taste like manna from heaven. So *grit it out* and reap the rewards for the rest of the day.

SATURDAY

Longer run for an hour (about 5 miles) at your normal pace. You are working on extending the length of your easy run while maintaining the same speed—to get you used to covering longer distances and give you plenty of practice for race day.

SUNDAY

Forty-five minutes of easy running. This should be a breeze for you now that you've done possibly your first-ever interval or hill session. It is amazing how the interval and hill training affect your fitness very quickly, making your "easy" run really seem just that—EASY.

A *Grit Doctor* REMINDER

DO NOT IGNORE your rest days. No matter what your mother tells you, you are not Superman. Your muscles need rest to repair and restore themselves, enabling you to improve and stretch them thereafter.

WEEK 2

MONDAY: Do some squats, try that Pilates class after all, pick up a jump rope—like last Monday, be active, just don't run.

TUESDAY: As per Week 1, warm up, then run for ten minutes, then do at least 5 x 100 meters (fast, slow, fast, slow, fast).

WEDNESDAY: As per Week 1, do your usual "easy" run.

THURSDAY: As per Week 1, do the same thing you did Tuesday, but do at least 5 x 100 meters and/or move a bit faster up that hill.

FRIDAY: REST.

SATURDAY: Long run—5.5 miles.

SUNDAY: As per Week 1, take it easy for 45 minutes.

WEEK 3

MONDAY: Again, do some interesting exercise other than running.

TUESDAY: As per Week 1, but at least 6 x 100 meters (fast, slow, fast, slow, fast, slow).

WEDNESDAY: As per Week 1.

THURSDAY: As per Week 1, but at least 6 x 100 meters and/or push yourself harder up that hill.

FRIDAY: REST.

SATURDAY: Long run—6 miles.

SUNDAY: As per Week 1.

WEEK 4

MONDAY: Exercise other than running, as per Week 1.

TUESDAY: As per Week 1, but at least 7 x 100 meters (fast, slow, fast, slow, fast, slow, fast).

WEDNESDAY: As per Week 1.

THURSDAY: As per Week 1, but at least 7 x 100 meters and/or push yourself harder up the hill.

FRIDAY: REST.

SATURDAY: Long run—7 miles.

SUNDAY: As per Week 1.

WEEK 5

MONDAY: Exercise other than running, as per Week 1.

THE GRIT DOCTOR'S 10K TRAINING PLAN

TUESDAY: As per Week 1, but at least 8 x 100 meters (fast, slow, fast, slow, fast, slow, fast, slow).

WEDNESDAY: As per Week 1.

THURSDAY: As per Week 1, but at least 8 x 100 meters and/or really *nail* that hill.

FRIDAY: REST.

SATURDAY: Long run—8 miles.

SUNDAY: As per Week 1.

WEEK 6

MONDAY: Exercise other than running, as per Week 1.

TUESDAY: As per Week 1, but 7 x 100 meters.

WEDNESDAY: As per Week 1.

THURSDAY: As per Week 1, but 7 x 100 meters and/or run fast up that hill.

FRIDAY: REST.

SATURDAY: Long run—8 miles.

SUNDAY: As per Week 1.

WEEK 7

MONDAY: REST.

TUESDAY: As per Week 1, but 5 x 100 meters and really push yourself on the fast laps.

WEDNESDAY: As per Week 1.

THURSDAY: As per Week 1, but 5 x 100 meters and really go for it on the fast laps and/or the hill.

FRIDAY: REST.

SATURDAY: Long run—6 miles.

SUNDAY: As per Week 1.

WEEK 8

MONDAY: REST.

TUESDAY: As per Week 1—4 x 100 meters.

WEDNESDAY: REST.

THURSDAY: As per Week 1—4 x 100 meters or take on a gentle hill.

FRIDAY: REST.

SATURDAY: RACE DAY. Good luck—may the grit be with you.

SUNDAY: SLEEP, EAT, AND DRINK A LOT (of water, too)!

The Final Word

Running makes you happy. . . .

Physiologically, running makes you happy because it stimulates the release of endorphins and encourages the production of serotonin, the same hormones that are released when you fall in love, gorge on chocolate, or have an orgasm. This happens both during the run and for a considerable time afterward. You will feel a sense of contentment and well-being known as a "runner's high."

You will also be happy because you look so much better than all of your non-running contemporaries—and both you and they know it. Guard against appearing smug about this in front of anyone whom you actually like.

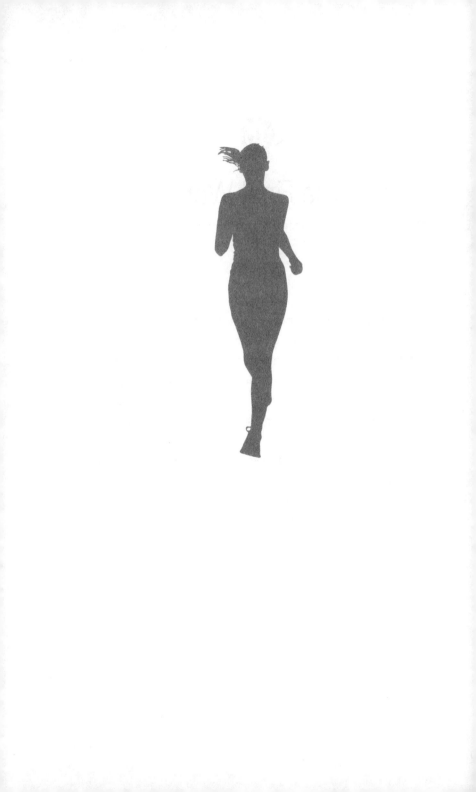

If you take only three things from this book, let it be these:

- Run.
- Drink more water.
- Eat less crap.

You. Can. Do. It.

Ruth . . .

I AM RIGHT there beside you, struggling to run. I had to start again from scratch—maybe not in terms of base fitness level, but mentally, I had to start from the beginning. I had zero motivation. Zero strength. Divorced from the voice of the Grit Doctor, I used every excuse in the book and added a new one: TWINS. Eight months later I had to accept it was just that—another excuse, one which could easily be on the list in Chapter 2 (page 42).

Whatever you have going on in your life that makes you think you are different from everyone else, it is nonsense. Get over it. We all have the same twenty-four hours. Singles, couples, fat dads, thin moms, young girls, old monks, deranged mothers of multiples. Put on your sneakers. Be all that you can be. Run.

Health and Safety

GENUINE INJURY

You *know* when you have a proper injury. How? Because you are in agony. If you sprain an ankle or have strained a muscle, you won't be able to walk on it, let alone run. Get home and immediately apply an ice pack wrapped in a dish towel to the injured area. (Frozen peas are perfect, and you will, of course, have a stash in your freezer because of your newfound love of green vegetables.) Don't give yourself a further injury or freeze yourself to death by holding it on for too long. Then bandage the affected area firmly and elevate it (the injured part of your body should be raised above your heart) to help reduce swelling. For anything more serious than a sprain or strain, go to the doctor and, if necessary, get a referral to a physical therapist. And for goodness' sake, follow their instructions.

Ruth . . .

WHEN I WENT for that first run after having the twins and hurting my knee, I did a very stupid thing indeed. I'd had a pain in my knee for a few days before I went running, but I told myself it was nothing, and I went anyway. I also knew that the pain would probably disappear after a few minutes because all the hormones released through running are very effective at masking aches and pains. Sure enough, ten minutes into the run I didn't feel any pain. But the relief from pain is very temporary. I woke up the next morning in agony and could not run for a long time afterward. And I had no one to blame but my own stupid self for not listening to my body. If you have pain in your knees, get it sorted out before running.

PREVENTION IS BETTER THAN CURE

Don't run on concrete if you can avoid it, and certainly not until after you have invested in proper running shoes—these two things are your best insurance policy against injury and will help you to avoid the most common running complaints. The shoes will support your feet and ankles properly and help cushion your knees from the impact of running, which is exacerbated by running on a hard surface. While wearing the correct shoes, always warm up through walking and swinging your arms for 10 minutes first, and try your best to stick to grass, trails, and tracks as much as possible. Rest is also important, but there's no need to overdo it. Those on my program are getting plenty of rest anyway, so don't worry about it. If, however, you have become a running nut and are nailing it six days a week, you **must have a rest day** and listen to your body.

GET OFF YOUR ASS AND RUN!   #gritdoctor

GENERAL SAFETY

- Don't get so into your run that you try to cross roads when pedestrian traffic lights are red. Jog in place until they turn green.
- Be aware that running on a road with an iPod is potentially risky as you can't hear approaching traffic or ax-wielding psychos. If you're running through a busy area, or any area where you feel even a smidge uncomfortable, turn the music *down*.
- If you must run on a road, please run against the direction of traffic, so you can see cars coming.
- Avoid running in deserted areas, especially at night.
- Ideally, stick to well-lit, populated areas while running.
- Always carry identification in case of an accident.
- Use proper sun protection (I have terrible sunspots from running without shades, hat, or sunscreen). Also, try to avoid running during the hottest part of the day (noon to 3 PM) during the summer or while on vacation.
- You can do yourself more harm than good by wearing knee or ankle supports without medical advice. You are most likely using them as a psychological crutch (for which the Grit Doctor has no time) and may actually be causing yourself damage in the process. Get the problem sorted by going to see your doctor and getting a referral to a physical therapist, an osteopath, or a podiatrist if necessary and getting the injury treated. You are not able to diagnose a knee or ankle injury yourself, nor, sadly, is the Grit Doctor.

- Wear orthotics (special shoe inserts) if you have very odd feet—the assistant at the running store will advise you on this.
- If you're a woman, run wearing a sports bra appropriate for the high-impact activity that running is.
- Make yourself visible to passing traffic if you are running in the dark by making yourself look like a crossing guard in light-reflective clothes—a reflective strip that goes across your front and back is ideal.

Online Resources for Runners

THE *grit doctor* SAYS

THE GRIT DOCTOR is not a big fan of the Internet. In the time it takes for you to Google what you were initially interested in—and then Google something else that looks interesting but is entirely unrelated to your initial search—you could have been on a good 30-minute fat-busting run. That said, once you have caught the running bug, the Internet is a useful place to get you involved in racing, joining clubs, and shopping for gear.

For Racing and Running Clubs

runnersworld.com/race-finder
coolrunning.com
active.com

For Establishing Your Running Circuit

runningmap.com
mapmyrun.com
mapometer.com

Running-Specific Stretching Tips and Tutorials

livestrong.com/running-stretches

youtube.com/watch?v=LmBp05_DMrQ

Shoe Shops and Other Shops for Runners

roadrunnersports.com

runyourcity.com

runnersworld.com/store-finder

titlenine.com

A *Grit Doctor* FASHION TIP FOR THE LADIES

BE SURE TO buy your first running sports bra in a shop. Your sports bra size may be different from your usual bra size, and the shape and feel is certainly different—it's snugger, to minimize movement and prevent injury. It really will pay to try a few on (like the shoes) before you make up your mind. Once you have got the knack, know your size and what works best for you, save yourself the time and buy them online. The time you save shopping can be spent running.

Ruth . . .

THE GRIT DOCTOR has been forced to become better friends with the Internet since writing this book, and you might like to check out my blog at gritdoctor.wordpress.com for updates on my running adventures and the occasional bout of Grit Doctor wisdom. Or follow me on Twitter @gritdoctor and use the hashtag #gritdoctor to discuss the book. Not my idea, but one forced upon me by my editor.

Running Log

WEEK 1

	DAY	TASK	NOTES
☐	Monday	Read Step 1 (page 50) Walk 3- to 4-mile route	
☐	Tuesday	REST	
☐	Wednesday	Read Step 2 (page 52) Repeat Monday	
☐	Thursday	Read Step 3 (page 52) Repeat Monday, increase pace	
☐	Friday	REST	
☐	Saturday	Read Step 4 (page 54) Begin as on Thursday. Walk first 10 minutes, jog *slowly* for 5, walk remainder	
☐	Sunday	Repeat Saturday	

WEEK 2

	DAY	TASK	NOTES
☐	Monday	REST	
☐	Tuesday	Walk first 10 minutes, jog *slowly* for 5, walk remainder	
☐	Wednesday	Repeat Tuesday, but extend *slow* jog to 10 minutes	
☐	Thursday	Repeat Wednesday	
☐	Friday	REST	
☐	Saturday	Repeat Thursday	
☐	Sunday	Repeat Saturday	

WEEK 3

Ten-minute walk to warm up, followed by 15 minutes of incredibly slow jogging, followed by walking for the remainder of the circuit without stopping. Two rest days of your choice, but not consecutive to one another. Plan out your week in advance here.

	DAY	TASK	NOTES
☐	Monday		
☐	Tuesday		
☐	Wednesday		
☐	Thursday		
☐	Friday		
☐	Saturday		
☐	Sunday		

#griddoctor

GET OFF YOUR ASS AND RUN!

WEEK 4

Ten-minute walk to warm up, followed by 20 minutes of jogging (slow down the pace of the jog if necessary to sustain it for 20 minutes), followed by walking the remainder of the circuit without stopping. Two rest days, but not on consecutive days. Plan out your week in advance here.

	DAY	TASK	NOTES
☐	Monday		
☐	Tuesday		
☐	Wednesday		
☐	Thursday		
☐	Friday		
☐	Saturday		
☐	Sunday		

WEEK 5

Ten-minute walk to warm up, followed by 20 minutes of jogging (slow down the pace of the jog if necessary to sustain it for 20 minutes), followed by walking the remainder of the circuit without stopping. Two rest days, but not on consecutive days. Plan out your week in advance here.

	DAY	TASK	NOTES
☐	Monday		
☐	Tuesday		
☐	Wednesday		
☐	Thursday		
☐	Friday		
☐	Saturday		
☐	Sunday		

#gritdoctor

GET OFF YOUR ASS AND RUN!

WEEK 6

Ten-minute walk to warm up, followed by 30 minutes of *very slow* jogging, followed by walking the remainder of the circuit without stopping. Two rest days, but not on consecutive days. Plan out your week in advance here.

	DAY	TASK	NOTES
☐	Monday		
☐	Tuesday		
☐	Wednesday		
☐	Thursday		
☐	Friday		
☐	Saturday		
☐	Sunday		

WEEK 7

Ten-minute walk to warm up, followed by 35 minutes of *very slow* jogging, followed by walking what remains of the circuit without stopping. Two rest days, but not on consecutive days. Plan out your week in advance here.

	DAY	TASK	NOTES
☐	Monday		
☐	Tuesday		
☐	Wednesday		
☐	Thursday		
☐	Friday		
☐	Saturday		
☐	Sunday		

WEEK 8

Ten-minute walk to warm up, followed by 40 minutes of *very slow* jogging, followed by walking home if there is anything left of the circuit. If not, always cool down by walking a few hundred meters before you go back indoors. Two rest days, but not on consecutive days. Read and observe Step 5 (page 59). Plan out your week in advance here.

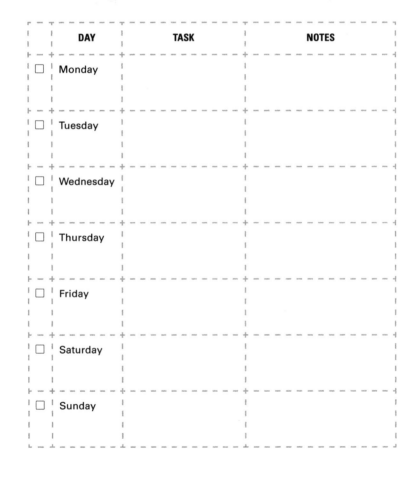

	DAY	TASK	NOTES
☐	Monday		
☐	Tuesday		
☐	Wednesday		
☐	Thursday		
☐	Friday		
☐	Saturday		
☐	Sunday		

GET OFF YOUR ASS AND RUN! #gritdoctor

The Grit Doctor's
Ultimate Running Playlist

The Grit Doctor prefers to run in Zen-like silence, but if you (like Olly) need thumping bass lines or cheesy '80s power ballads to get you going, try making your own running playlist and using it to spur yourself on. Here are some suggestions.

For those who prefer a very literal running soundtrack:

"Run the World (Girls)"	Beyoncé
"Born to Run"	Bruce Springsteen
"Young Hearts Run Free"	Candi Staton
"Band on the Run"	Wings
"Running Up That Hill"	Kate Bush
"Run to You"	Bryan Adams
"Run This Town"	Jay-Z, featuring Kanye West and Rihanna
"Shoot the Runner"	Kasabian
"Run to the Hills"	Iron Maiden
"100 Miles and Runnin'"	N.W.A.
"I'm Gonna Be (500 Miles)"	The Proclaimers
"Run"	Snow Patrol
"Running to Stand Still"	U2

And, of course . . .

"Chariots of Fire"	Vangelis
"Eye of the Tiger"	Survivor

In a survey of fellow runners, an eclectic mix of tunes came to light, ranging from hip(ish) to deeply uncool (some of which are Grit Doctor faves for cutting shapes on the dance floor*). In no particular order:

"Bonkers"	Dizzee Rascal
(for the adrenaline rush)	
"Rolling in the Deep"	Adele
"Dog Days Are Over"	Florence and the Machine
"Sex on Fire"*	Kings of Leon
(I understand this is also the technical name for the symptoms runners can experience if they wear the wrong kind of shorts)	
"I Need a Dollar"	Aloe Blacc
"Common People"*	Pulp
"More Than a Feeling"	Boston
"I Need a Hero"	Bonnie Tyler
"Don't Stop Believin'"	Journey
(but it was ruined for me by Glee . . .)	
"We Built This City"	Starship
"Love Shack"	The B-52's
"Together in Electric Dreams"*	Philip Oakey and Giorgio Moroder

"Little Lovin'"	Lissie
(for the lyric "Why you runnin'?,"	
which always makes me smile	
when the burn kicks in)	
"Apache"	Incredible Bongo Band
"I Was Drunk"	Riva Starr, featuring
(very motivating . . . somehow)	Nôze
"Time to Pretend"	MGMT
"Make Me Smile	Steve Harley and
(Come Up and See Me)"	Cockney Rebel

#gritdoctor

GET OFF YOUR ASS AND RUN!

Acknowledgments

In no particular order: My husband, Olly, for his brilliant ideas and for humoring me. Our sons, Sebastian and Rufus (not sure for what yet). For early encouragement: Joan Johnson (1917–2010), Sacha Bonsor, Alice Lutyens, Veronique Jackson, Adam Morane-Griffiths, and Louise and Roger Lamberth. All the contributors: Charlotte Pilain, Laetitia Maklouf, Jane Davies, Alice Crawford, Toby Lisle and Nicola Fister (you know who you are), Barney and Louise Oswald, Father Henry Wansbrough OSB, Chris Spira, and Polly Whitton. My family: Mum and Dad, Auntie Bernadette, Pippa and Roger (for unending support and help with the twins), Simon, Peter (for the word *grit*), Anna, Matthew, and Jex. Merialeen and Lucie for looking after the twins, Sable D'Or, Café Nero, Nyborgs and Feast in Muswell Hill for allowing me to make one skinny cappuccino (and the odd pain au raisin) last a whole day while writing.

My wonderful agents, Alice Saunders and Abigail Koons (without whom none of this would be happening), Hannah Boursnell and Rhiannon Smith of Little, Brown, for their faith and mastery. And most important, to everyone at The Experiment, but particularly my extraordinary editor, Cara Bedick, and assistant managing editor, Molly Cavanaugh, for their hard work and commitment and for embracing the spirit of the Grit Doctor so wholeheartedly.

About the Author

RUTH FIELD is a trial attorney and passionate runner who, while pregnant and under doctor's orders not to run, decided to write *Get Off Your Ass and Run!* as an outlet for her frustration. She lives in North London with her husband and twin sons. She has a fitness and motivation column in the *Irish Times* and has been featured in the *Globe and Mail* among other publications.

IF YOU'VE BEEN INSPIRED BY THE GRIT
DOCTOR, GET IN TOUCH AND LET HER
KNOW ABOUT IT.

Twitter
@gritdoctor
#gritdoctor

Facebook
facebook.com/thegritdoctor

The Grit Doctor's Blog
gritdoctor.wordpress.com